THE ESSENTIAL FAMILY GUIDE TO CARING FOR OLDER PEOPLE

Deborah Stone

GREEN TREE
LONDON • OXFORD • NEW YORK • NEW DELHI • SYDNEY

GREEN TREE
Bloomsbury Publishing Plc
50 Bedford Square, London, WC1B 3DP, UK

BLOOMSBURY, GREEN TREE and the Green Tree logo are trademarks of Bloomsbury Publishing Plc

First published in Great Britain 2019

A catalogue record for this book is available from the British Library

Library of Congress Cataloguing-in-Publication data has been applied for

ISBN: TPB: 978-1-4729-6543-1; eBook: 978-1-4729-6542-4

2 4 6 8 10 9 7 5 3 1

Typeset in Minion Pro by Deanta Global Publishing Services, Chennai, India
Printed and bound in Great Britain by CPI Group (UK) Ltd., Croydon, CR0 4YY

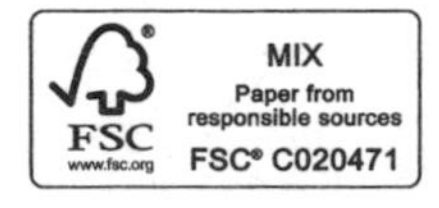

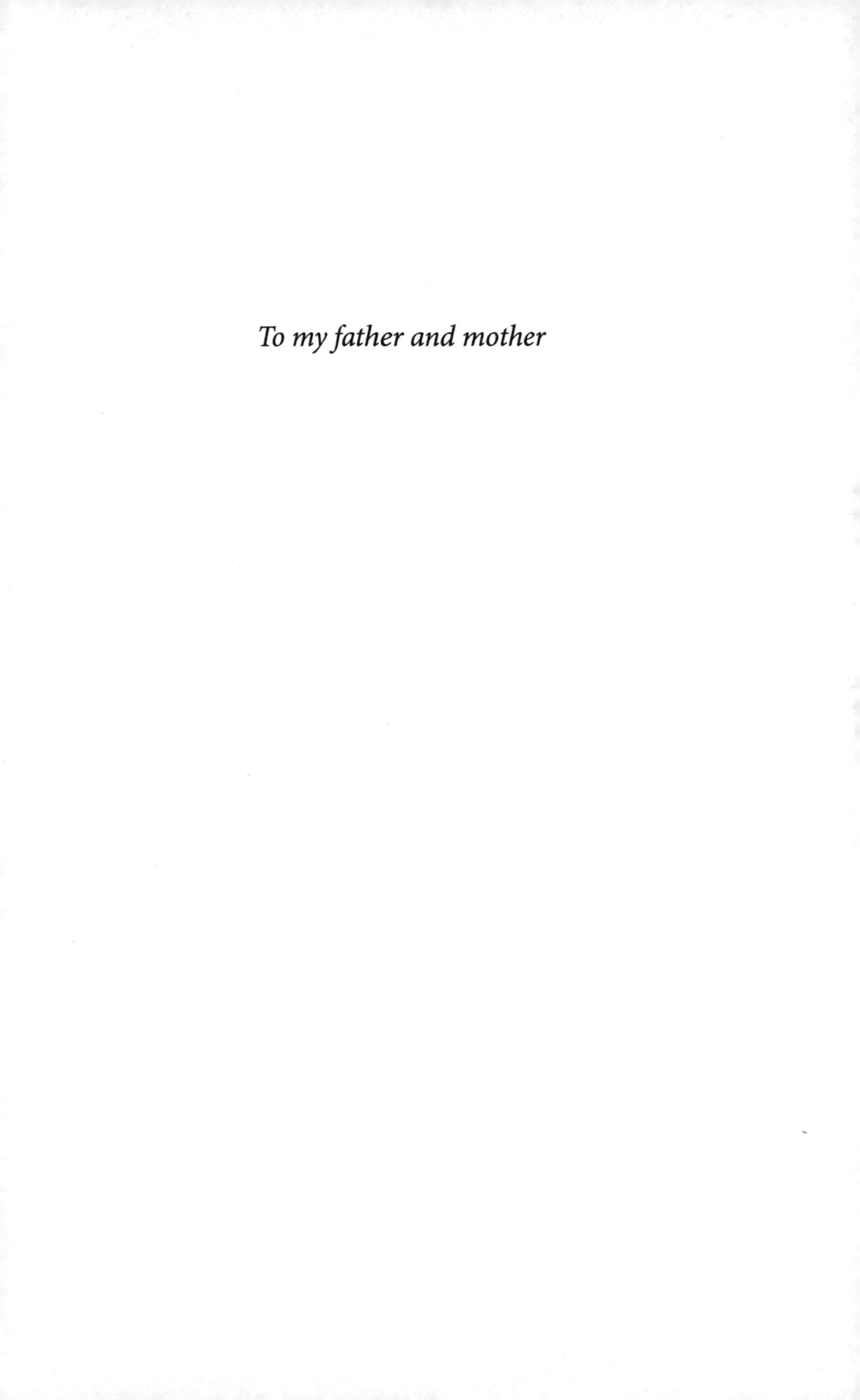

To my father and mother

Contents

Foreword

Caring for someone we love as they get older and become less independent is one of the most emotionally and physically challenging things that anyone will ever have to do.

This task is made all the more difficult because it is sometimes thrust upon us by a sudden event, such as a stroke, a fall, or the diagnosis of a long-term condition, and – when we are at our most vulnerable and are emotionally fragile – the system makes things worse by its complexity, and the seemingly impenetrable bureaucracy that surrounds it.

Many people come to this strange new world of health and social care without any experience of how to navigate the system, and with no knowledge of what questions to ask, or what choices to make.

Deborah Stone was faced with this scenario and has used the experience of supporting her parents to help and support other people going through similar challenges.

The Essential Family Guide to Caring for Older People is a clear, simple guide to a very complex process. All aspects of supporting older people are to be found in this incredibly comprehensive and useful publication.

This book is a practical guide to steering a course through a health and social care system that is increasingly focused on trying to stop older people getting services. What I find particularly useful is that the book can be used in every step of the journey. It covers clearly and comprehensively the assessment system, how you make informed choices about what care services to use and the responsibilities of local government, the NHS and the individual. All are clearly outlined and the book can be used as a reference manual as you move through the different choices you have to make.

One of the important aspects of this book is that it was written by somebody who has had practical experience of the challenges of supporting someone you love. As well as being a guide to the system, it helps people to understand that they are not alone, and Deborah shares her knowledge and experience in a way that gives practical help, and better understanding of the emotional challenges of caring.

I hope that anybody who has older relatives will read this, as it will enable you to navigate a complex system with much greater ease and deliver better outcomes for the people you love and all those who care for them.

Professor Martin Green OBE
Chief Executive: Care England
Chair: The International Longevity Centre-UK

A Note From the Author

I understand what it is like to care for an older relative. My father suffered from vascular dementia for over eight years and my family and I struggled to find the right information and care to help him. At the same time, I was running my own business, my husband travelled a great deal and I had two young children to look after, as well as running my home. I was constantly stressed, and often ill as a result.

My mother is still alive and has lived alone now for 16 years, but suffers from a range of complicated ailments and is barely able to walk. There are often emergency hospital admissions and unforeseen crises to deal with, which have ranged from drinking surgical spirit and potassium permanganate instead of cough mixture on two separate occasions to getting stuck in the shower one morning and breaking her pelvis in three places as she tried to open the door. There are some even more gruesome examples, which I have decided to spare you.

How I would have loved to have had a manual to guide me through the minefield of caring for my relatives, both now and earlier; one which covered all of the main issues I needed to know about, and which could have pointed me in the right direction to obtain further information. More importantly, I would have liked something that might have reassured me that I was doing my best, even when, quite often, I really felt that I was failing. But it did not exist, so I decided to write one – and here it is! So I do hope that you will find this book useful as a guide to help you care for your older relatives.

I have written this book for family carers of older people, but it is just as useful for you if you are an older person yourself. Carers range widely in age from people in their 40s, right through to their 90s.

They can be sons, daughters, nieces, nephews and very often, spouses and partners.

These days it is hard to define what 'older' actually means, as so many people look and feel great well into their 70s, 80s and 90s. The official statistics, however, define 'older' as post-pensionable age, i.e. 65+, and then make a further distinction above the age of 80. I hope that whatever your age and circumstances, you will find this book an invaluable resource to help you through the later life challenges we all face. It will guide you through the essential elements of planning ahead for financing care, sorting out legal issues and reviewing care options, as well as providing many helpful tips and suggestions about living a full and happy later life, as well as what to do when ill health and crises strike.

How to use this book

This book is a manual for you to use as often as you need to. You can dip in and out of it, depending on what information and advice you are looking for. If you do read it from cover to cover, you may find that some topics arise more than once, such as care assessments or certain family issues, but this is because particular sections demand that these issues be discussed as part of that particular topic. However, in other instances, the book will direct you to another page for fuller details on a subject, which might be mentioned in passing at a particular point in the book. If in doubt, you can find references to everything in the index.

Introduction

Our population is ageing faster every year and, as a result, more and more of us are caring for older family members. Currently, around 18 per cent of people in the UK are aged 65 and over, and 3 per cent are aged 85 and over. In eight years' time, one fifth of the UK population will be aged 65 or over, and this will rise to a quarter of the total population (19 million people) by 2045. The overall percentage of people over 80 is also growing rapidly and will see a fourfold increase in the 50 years from 2000 to 2050. The United Nations estimates that, by 2050, the over-80 age group will number almost 379 million worldwide, about 5.5 times as many as in 2000. By way of comparison, in 1950, there were fewer than 14 million people aged over 80 worldwide.

While it is good news that people are generally living longer, unfortunately many people live longer in ill health, often coping with a number of different illnesses and ailments. This places enormous stress in terms of time, money and emotional commitment on the millions of carers who help them. There are around 11 million direct and indirect carers in the UK and three in every five people will be carers at some point in their lives. One in five people aged between 50 and 64 are carers in the UK. Forty-two per cent of carers are men and 58 per cent are women. The current economic value of the contribution made by carers in the UK is £132 billion a year. By 2030, the number of carers will increase by 3.4 million. Many people are caring for someone with dementia. There are currently 800,000 people living with dementia in the UK, with 670,000 unpaid carers looking after them.

Sixty-five per cent of older carers – those aged between 60 and 94 – have long-term health problems, or a disability themselves and 69 per cent of older carers say that being a carer has an adverse effect on their own mental health. One third of older carers say they have cancelled treatment or an operation for themselves – according to a survey by the Carers Trust – and lack of respite care, or other forms of support, can have very serious consequences for carers, with many experiencing both physical and mental ill health. Carers providing more than 50 hours of care per week are twice as likely to report health problems as the average population. For example, carers providing high levels of care were associated with a 23 per cent higher risk of stroke. Caring also carries a financial burden. Fifty-three per cent of carers have borrowed money as a result of their caring responsibilities and 60 per cent have used all of their savings to cover the costs of caring. Twenty-three per cent have either re-mortgaged their home, or downsized to a smaller property due to their caring responsibilities.

So we already face a major challenge with regard to elder care and that challenge grows larger every day. Yet just 23 per cent of adults with living relatives* say they have already discussed future care arrangements with their relatives and a third of people in later life have no idea how they would pay for any future care needs. For many of us, discussing future care wishes, options and how to pay for them is a subject which is avoided until a crisis hits … and then it is often too late. Most people are unaware of the financial restrictions relating to paying for care – which in effect means that most people have to fund their own care in the UK – or of the necessary legal considerations we should all arrange well in advance of declining health. Discussing preferred care options and how to fund them well ahead of a crisis can make the caring role much easier when the time comes.

* Polled by YouGov for Carers Trust, 2015

This book aims to offer information, help and advice to all families, whether they are currently caring for older relatives, a spouse or partner, or just starting to plan ahead for the future. It will offer advice on all aspects of caring for an older person, or help you if you are getting older yourself and want to start planning ahead.

CHAPTER ONE

What to Do If You Need Help NOW

If you need to get urgent help for an older relative or relative now, this is where to start.

Go to see the GP first

Your older relative's GP should be your first port of call if you are concerned about their health and ability to cope at home. The GP will run tests if necessary and will do two main things:

- Discuss medical treatment and arrange any further tests they may require
- Liaise with the local authority to get a care assessment for your relative.

Managing a care assessment

Care assessments are carried out at home. It is very helpful to write down any important points before the assessment, so you can input your concerns and do not forget any issues you want to raise. The care assessment will look at your relative's needs and recommend the appropriate services. Normally, an assessment is required before any services can be provided by the social services department of a local authority, but if the need is urgent, the local authority can provide help without carrying out the assessment, following discussion with your relative's GP. The local authority will implement a community care assessment in order to ascertain whether a person needs a community care service and, if they do, whether it can be provided by the local authority. The assessment should provide certain basic information and a care plan should be drawn up. A wide range of services could be needed, from mobility aids and adaptations in the person's own home to the provision of care workers, or placing your relative in residential care. You can read the full details about care assessments and what they entail on pages 70–73.

Care options

There is a range of care options available, depending on the results of the assessment. It might be that your relative can remain at home, but will need help with adaptations and some form of live-in care, for example.

Personal budgets

The local authority will give your elderly relative a *personal budget* to manage to pay for their care, depending on their entitlement. You can find full details on personal budgets on page 51.

At home care

If you are employing carers, it is also very important to vet them properly and to ask the right questions. You can see a list of recommended questions to ask on pages 76–77.

Care homes

The care assessment may conclude that your relative needs to move into a care home. If this is the case, the local authority will advise you of the options available. Care homes differ depending on need, ranging from residential housing with a warden to nursing homes and dementia care. You can read about the different types of care homes available on pages 84–85.

It is essential to visit any care home before you agree to place your relative there. There are several things to look out for and you can read about the best tests of a good care home on pages 85–87. You should also check out any home with the Care Quality Commission's rating service at www.cqc.org.uk.

Caring from a distance

Many people live a long distance away from their elderly relative and this can be very challenging in terms of providing care. However, there are things you can do to alleviate some of this stress, including utilising technology to improve communication. There are several recommendations on what to do when living a distance away from your relative on pages 89–92.

Carer assessments

Caring for a relative can be exhausting. You can ask your local authority for a carer's assessment for yourself to help you manage. You can read more about carer assessments on pages 70–73. You should also think about respite care to give yourself a break occasionally and you can talk to your local authority about this as part of your own carer's assessment.

Funding care

Care can be extremely expensive, especially as the cap on care costs is low. Ideally, you should think about how to fund care before a crisis hits, but if not, there are a number of options to consider, which you can read about in more detail in Chapter 5, pages 45–48.

Sorting out the legal issues

If your relative is becoming frail, it is sensible to consider getting Legal Power of Attorney (LPA) over them in order to help them with their legal, financial and medical affairs. Without this, it is difficult to help them with their personal finances and medical wishes. You can find out more about LPA on pages 36–40. Also, you must ensure your relative has made a will, as if they die intestate (without a will), most of what they leave will go to the government. You can learn more about how and why to make a will in Chapter 4, pages 27–32.

CHAPTER TWO

How to Cope as a Carer

The sandwich generation

As more of us have children later, in our 30s and 40s, we often don't think about the consequences of this decision 15 years or so down the line with regard to elder care. As a result, many of us find that we have the tricky challenge of bringing up teenagers at the same time as having to look after older relatives. As many of us know, bringing up teenagers is challenging – the constant bargaining, the sulking, the negotiating, the worry … need I go on? You need to be around for them as much as when they were smaller, but in a different way and it can be draining, emotionally and physically. If you add into this the fact that you and your partner have hit middle age and that your relatives may well be older and less able to cope than before, you are suddenly dealing with many stressful dynamics all at once.

Distance can be a big problem. Often relatives do not live close by and the strain of long-distance care can really start to tell. Distance care can also lead to tension among siblings, as one sibling takes on the lion's share of the caring responsibilities if they live closest. The child who lives closer to their relatives can start to resent the sibling who lives too far away to be there every day. The sibling who lives further away can feel constantly guilty and find it difficult to make the journeys as often as they would like, due to time and money constraints. It is really important to talk about this between you and your siblings, so that everyone can discuss how they can help in the best way, given their individual circumstances. Try to work it out between you sensibly and without recriminations.

It is worth saying a little more about sibling rivalry, which can intensify as adult children vie, one last time, for a relative's love or financial support. Even as relatives grow dependent on children, their desire to cling to old, familiar roles can create a dysfunctional mess. It is crucial for families to work out how to care for their older relative together and to work through any differences they may have. If they do not, their relatives will suffer – and so will the siblings. Try to put past difficulties or current resentments to one side and discuss what is best for your relative. If you have fallen out with your sibling in the past, try to give them another chance, but be realistic about what they will and will not do – and what you will and will not do. Agree what needs to be done for your relative and share out the roles according to distance, time and, as far as you can, fairness. Talk regularly and openly about the situation. Do not bottle up your resentment, as this will not help you, your siblings or your relative. You can lend support from a distance if you do not live close by, by dealing with financial and other administrative affairs. Siblings living closer to their relative and dealing with more day-to-day care will be stressed and tired. They need understanding. This should not make you feel guilty. Keep in touch with each other and your relative by phone, text, Skype, FaceTime and email as much as you can.

Alice lived a few minutes' drive away from her mother and father in Manchester, but her sister Jane lived in London. Her mother was housebound with rheumatoid arthritis and her father was in the early stages of dementia. Alice began to spend increasing amounts of time with her parents, helping them with shopping, cooking, cleaning and dressing. She did not work, but had a teenage family to look after and a husband. She called her sister Jane regularly to inform her of the problems their parents were suffering and the time it was taking her to care for them, but she felt that Jane never really listened and always used the excuse of being too far away to be able to help. After all, Jane had an important job, while Alice didn't work and Alice was closer and had more time. It was also expensive and time-consuming to keep dashing to Manchester every weekend. Resentment between the sisters grew and they never took the time to sit down together to thrash out the problems and to agree how each of them could help the other. The situation deteriorated over the next couple of years, with frequent, hostile exchanges taking place between the sisters. The result was that, after their parents died, the sisters rarely spoke again.

It can be very difficult to balance your time between your own family and elder care, but try to remember that it is important to understand that, while you obviously do have an enormous responsibility for your relatives, you also have responsibilities towards your partner and to your children, if you have them, and that you cannot do it all. Recognise that sometimes you need to get external help and do not feel guilty about it. Everyone has very busy lives and you need to be organised to keep on top of the demands of older relatives, your children and still ensure that you have some time for yourself and your partner. It is also important to look after your own health otherwise you will be unable to help look after anyone at all. Keep a diary of who is doing what and when, and explain to your children, if they're old enough, that you need their help with managing the situation. Believe it or not, sometimes the kids, even at quite a young age, can help with your relatives. They can visit them, chat to them over the phone or via Skype, watch TV with them, teach them how to use a computer or iPad, or play a card game with them. They can also do some jobs for your relatives to lighten the load.

It is so important to ask for support when you feel you need it. Meet your relative's GP and discuss their needs, ideally with your sibling(s), and if this is not possible, agree what you need to discuss beforehand and debrief each other afterwards. You can make an appointment with your relative's doctor, but the doctor cannot discuss your relative's confidential records without their permission, or unless you hold legal power of attorney (see pages 36–40 for more details.) You can, however, make your relative's doctor aware of the problems your relative is facing and encourage the doctor to make contact with them, either at the surgery, or on a home visit.

Ask the doctor for care support and assessments as needed. Remember to keep your relative's welfare paramount. If you are struggling to see eye to eye with your sibling(s), get an independent neighbour, friend or GP to help mediate. Above all, try to keep a sense of humour as much as you can. Remember, you are not alone. Millions of people in the UK are dealing with the same issues as you every single day.

Looking after yourself as a carer

Being a carer can be hard work – physically, mentally and emotionally. Fortunately, there is a great deal of support out there for people who find themselves in a caring role. It is vitally important that carers are able to get timely advice, tailored to their individual circumstances and accessible in a way that suits their particular situation and fortunately, there are a number of ways in which you can access help.

Online communities and forums offer a community of other carers, who also understand the impact that caring for a family member or friend can have. Carers have the opportunity to talk to one another and get vital support. Forums and discussion boards are a great opportunity to ask questions about anything related to caring. You might have a question about different forms of assessment, or how to negotiate with health and social care professionals. Or you may want to offload some of your worries or concerns, or share something good that has happened. Discussion boards and forums cover a wide range of subjects and have an equally diverse range of people replying to and interacting with each other.

A chatroom provides the opportunity to meet with other carers. Some of the conversation is related to caring, but it also allows you the chance to socialise with others without having to leave the house, which can be difficult for carers. Joining a chatroom is really straightforward once you have registered.

Local carer centres across the country offer practical, as well as emotional, support to people caring for a family member or friend, who would otherwise not be able to cope. Carer centres are usually run by independent charities and offer great opportunities for carers to get together, share their experiences and support each other. A regular get together can be a great opportunity to meet with other people who understand the impact that being a carer can have. Sometimes, it is really important to be able to speak to someone who understands what you are going through and has been in a similar situation themselves. All carers are welcome and you can find your local services by searching for 'carers' centre' in your area online.

It is essential that carers look after themselves in order to be able to continue to look after the person they care for. Carers' centres and schemes have staff who can provide respite opportunities so that carers can have a much-needed break. Having a chance to recuperate and rest and do something for *you* can make a real difference to your health and happiness. A little bit of 'me time' is not selfish, but often essential for the health and wellbeing of all concerned. Staff at carers centres have specialised knowledge of the benefits system and how it relates to being a carer and are able to help with making sure that carers are claiming for all of the financial support to which they are entitled. They can help you to navigate your way through assessment processes in order to access support available for statutory services and advocate on behalf of carers to secure support. You can also find a great deal of support and advice at Carers UK www.carersuk.org and the Carers Trust www.carers.org.

Felicity was exhausted from looking after her disabled father, her two young children and holding down her job. She started to suffer from bad bouts of bronchitis, which would recur every few weeks. Eventually, she got pneumonia and ended up in hospital for a month, unable to care for anyone. 'If I had just stood back a little and tried to get some respite care, I would not have become so ill myself, but I thought I was the only one who could do it and that asking for help meant I was a bad daughter. I felt guilty all the time … and then, when I got sick myself, I felt even worse. I was no use to anyone and my father died while I was in hospital. I never forgave myself.'

Local authorities have a duty to offer help to carers. They have to offer carer assessments, which consider offering additional help to make the caring role easier. Local authorities have the same responsibility to assess carers' needs as they do to assess those with care needs. They are required to look at how they can help carers in their role and how they can provide services and support which will benefit the carer. A carer's assessment is different from the community care assessment for the person in need of care. If you, as a carer, have your own need for community care services because of ill health or disability, you may also be eligible for your own community care assessment. One way to help ensure this is to ask for a carer's assessment alongside a community care assessment for your relative, to ensure that both the needs of the older person and the carer responsible for them are assessed simultaneously. However, you can also request a carer assessment separately to a care assessment for an older person, which you are entitled to ask for irrespective of whether the person you are caring for is being assessed. It also enables local authorities to provide carers with services in their own right, in addition to any services they may be providing for the person being cared for.

The assessments must consider whether the carer participates, or wishes to participate, in any work, education, training or leisure activity. This recognises that carers should be able to access the same opportunities as those without caring responsibilities. Although local authorities have a duty to carry out carers' assessments, whether or not they provide services is their decision. They do not have a duty to do so.

Local authorities can provide respite care and this may be beneficial to you and to the person you are looking after. In some areas, respite care is provided by your local authority as a result of an assessment of you as a carer. In other areas, access to respite care is provided through a community care assessment of the person you are looking after. Ideally, it is better if both parties are assessed. The local authority will consider what help you need and decide which community care services it will provide to help you.

You can find more information on assessments and your local authority/council at www.gov.uk.

If you have a complaint about your assessment, it is advisable to try and sort it out with the person you have contact with, such as the assessor or care manager. There may simply have been a failure in communication, or a misunderstanding that can be easily rectified. However, if this is not successful, there is a local authority complaints procedure. The local authority will explain how to use this. The complaints procedure might be useful if there are problems arranging an assessment, or there is an unreasonably long wait for an assessment. If the local authority complaints procedure does not resolve the issue either, you can take your complaint to the Local Government and Social Care Ombudsman at www.lgo.org.uk.

Coping as an older carer

The number of carers aged 85 and over has grown by 128 per cent in the last decade.[†] Many older carers provide vital care and support to their partners while letting their own health and wellbeing

[†]Carers UK and Age UK, 2015

deteriorate. They can also suffer enormous financial strain. Older people can be more reluctant to ask for, or to accept help, or even to identify themselves as a carer, as they may see it as a failure on their part, or worry that the person they are caring for will be taken away from them. They may also wish to remain independent for as long as possible. All of this can mean that older carers are unaware of the help they might be able to receive from their GP and social services. Hence, many older carers caring for a partner have to manage care for themselves and their partners, as well as running their home, which can result in high levels of stress and fatigue, especially when a carer is caring full-time and may be awake often in the night.

Audrey was married to Jim. When he got just past his 80th birthday, he started to show signs of dementia, which grew progressively worse. Audrey refused to get any help, insisting that she could look after Jim herself. Jim needed help with bathing and eating initially, but eventually, he was unable to walk or to use the toilet by himself. He often fell when Audrey was helping him out of bed, or getting him on or off the commode, because she could not take his weight and this led to multiple hospital admissions with broken bones and bruising. In the end, Audrey was admitted to hospital herself due to exhaustion and the family – none of whom lived close by – had to find emergency care for Jim while Audrey was treated in hospital. The family used this time to get a care assessment and the local authority provided help to the couple as a result once Audrey was discharged.

We should all try to be aware of older carers and the strains they are carrying within our communities. You might be one yourself, or you may be concerned about one of your relatives caring for the other. The right interventions to support the older carer may reduce the likelihood of increased future health, social care or residential care needs of both parties. Older carers can be socially isolated, which can cause depression and other mental health issues. Studies have shown how supporting carers, or providing them with a break, can improve their health, yet many older carers are unaware of their right to a carer's assessment and to respite care. If you are worried about your own situation, or that your own relatives, spouse or partner might be in this position, or you know of other older carers nearby, do talk to them about the options available and encourage them to contact their GP for help.

CHAPTER THREE

The Importance of Planning Ahead

Difficult conversations

It may be becoming apparent to you that your relative is coping less well than they used to, either physically or mentally. You want to help, yet sometimes it is not always easy to broach the subject with them for fear of wounding their pride and damaging their self-esteem. Often they will feel deeply concerned about their own loss of independence, yet it is important to have these conversations. So how can you raise these difficult issues?

It is a good idea to start by discussing the issues with your siblings or other members of the family to ensure you agree on the main problems, before discussing it with your relative. This might be about health issues, continuing to live alone, or management of their general finances and paperwork. Find out what the options are and how they might work before launching into any discussion with your relative. It is also essential to think about your relative's view as well as your own. If you think ahead about their possible objections, you can answer them calmly and knowledgeably. They may also have thought these issues through and have practical answers that you may not have thought of previously, so keep an open mind. Be prepared to revisit conversations several times and give your relative time to think on their own about your suggestions. If they feel under pressure, they are less likely to react positively. Most of us don't like change and it needs to be managed gradually. Try to talk in a relaxed environment, ideally without the kids running in and out, and where it is private enough to have a sensible conversation, and be prepared to listen and accept your relative's viewpoint.

Every situation varies. It can be that you are helping one relative to look after another older ailing relative, or that you have only one relative remaining. Whatever the case, you must consider certain issues, such as whether the person in question can manage certain day-to-day tasks. For example, can they still do the housework and their own cooking? Do they live alone and if so, can they cope? Are they carrying out caring duties for a partner and struggling? Can they manage the stairs? Do they appear nervous about living alone, or even as a couple, and can they still hear the door, the television and the phone? Do you think that they are feeling isolated or lonely, and are struggling to leave the house? Perhaps mobility is an issue, or their current home is simply too big to manage.

Based on these discussions, you can then address whether or not you should consider getting help. This might be help coming into their home and/or adapting their current home to assist them more easily. Maybe they should consider moving to a more manageable home in terms of size and/or location, or moving in with you, or with another relative. Alternatively, they can consider a number of alternative housing options, including sheltered accommodation, full residential care, or possibly a nursing home. Sometimes, your relative may not be well enough to participate in these conversations, but hopefully, they are, and if so, lay out all the pros and cons of each option, after having been through them yourself.

Should your relative live with you?

This is an option many people choose and often it works very well. Before making this decision, however, you need to assess this option carefully and consider a number of factors. Think about how it will affect your relationship with your partner and your family life with your children. Consider whether you have the time to take on this responsibility and all it entails, especially if your relative needs medical care and may need more in the future. Could you adapt your home if you needed to do so, both physically and financially?

You also need to ask your relative if they want to live with you, as they may be less keen on the idea than you are. In addition, they might be concerned about moving away from their friends and leaving behind local activities which they enjoy. It is not always easy to make new friendship groups when you are older.

If you decide that it is not the right thing to do to bring a relative to live with you, be honest with yourself about it and do not feel guilty. You have responsibilities to your partner and children, as well as to your relative, and you have to ensure that you do not fundamentally disturb those other relationships.

Helping your relative with their affairs

If your relative is increasingly finding it difficult to manage their own affairs, or has been ill, you may want to consider taking out Lasting Power of Attorney (LPA). Many people think this is a step only taken when someone is too ill to make their own decisions, but it is sensible to discuss taking this out on behalf of your relative before they become unable to cope. With soaring dementia rates (someone is diagnosed every three minutes in the UK), it is more important than ever for people to act while they are still mentally fit. It is highly recommended that people not only put their own power of attorney in place, but that they also support older relatives by helping them to get their affairs sorted out too.

There are two types of Lasting Power of Attorney (POA): health and finance. The health power of attorney means you can make medical decisions on behalf of your relative, should they be unable to do so. The financial power of attorney means that you can manage their financial affairs on their behalf, should they need you to do so. Often this is a big decision for a relative, as they fear giving up their own rights and control of their affairs. It can also lead to sibling conflict. It is often a good idea to hold joint power of attorney with siblings, so that decisions have to be made together and to avoid arguments. Be sensitive and be sensible on this issue. It is a very delicate one and should only be agreed upon at the right time for all parties, especially your relative. Remember that the actual power of attorney can only be used at such a time when your relative becomes incapacitated, regardless of when you have arranged it. Incapacity is decided by a doctor, who provides a letter to the relevant solicitor, informing them of your relative's incapacity and that they should put Lasting Power of Attorney into effect (see pages 23–24 and 36–40 for more on this).

Essential financial planning from 55 onwards

People are living longer, but unfortunately, many live for longer in ill health. Whereas a few years ago, someone might only need to be in a care home for a couple of years, now it can be a decade or longer. Whether you are lucky enough to live a long, healthy life, or you need care, getting older costs money so it is essential to think about finances as early as you can to ensure you have everything you need to live a comfortable life. A recent report revealed shockingly that 85 per cent of adults aged between 51 and 75 had done no financial planning for care in their old age.

Everyone beyond the age of 55 should begin to develop a financial checklist to see how healthy their finances are. After all, they might have to rely on them post-retirement for 30 years, or even longer. Everyone's circumstances are different, both financially and in terms of health and wellbeing, so it is very important to put together a realistic financial plan, which sets out both income and outgoings, not just for now, but over the next few years and decades, so you can work out what you have to live on and what you can save for future care.

It is a good idea to work out current monthly expenditure from bank statements and credit card statements and think about how this might change when you are not working, e.g. will you travel more? You can work out monthly income sources from pensions, bank interest and savings etc. Check what benefits you are entitled to, now and in the future, such as free bus travel and subsidised rail fares. You might be eligible for pension credits, which can top up the basic state pension, and you or your relative might also be eligible for other benefits, such as winter fuel payment.

If you have not already done so, you should decide when you want to retire, but remember that the state pension is not available until you reach the set pension age, which is between 61 and 68, depending when you were born and your gender (you can find out your exact situation at www.gov.uk). Anyone can carry on working past state pension age. If you do intend to retire, you need to give HMRC some notice, ideally a few months before. You also need to decide whether you want to delay drawing the state pension. Six months to a year before you intend to retire, you should contact your current and past pension providers and find out what pension is owed and how it will be paid. At work, you can contact the company's pension trustee to get this information. Regarding the state pension, the Pension Service should contact you four months before you retire, but you can call them instead on 0808 100 2658.

Main financial considerations when considering paying for care

It is a good idea to gather all financial information together. This could include bank statements, savings and investment statements, details of state pension and any benefits, such as attendance allowance (see pages 52–56 for more details). Check that all benefits are being claimed.

Help with this can be found at Citizens Advice, or on the government's website, www.gov.uk. Add up all the income and consider any expenses that will be ongoing. This should include all household and personal expenses. Look at the difference between income and expenditure and think about how this will change as your older relative ages. Consider what would happen if all care costs, either at home or in a care home, had to be paid for.

It is also essential to think about housing. Is it time to downsize to a smaller property and invest the excess in savings or care plans for the future? Does your relative want to consider moving to a property in a retirement community, which can meet their changing needs as they age? You might also consider the pros and cons of various types of savings for care, from deposit accounts to care fees annuities. You can read more on this in the section Financial Planning on page 45.

Essential legal planning for older people

There are a number of key legal documents, which are essential for you and your relative to have in place. In fact, anyone with a partner, spouse or offspring should ensure they have done their legal planning and agreed the main legal issues.

If you do not have a legal will, you cannot control to whom you can leave your estate. The only certainty of dying intestate (without a will) is that the tax man will be the main beneficiary. Wills are simple to make. You can do it yourself via the internet, or using shop-bought packs. You can also use a solicitor, or take advantages of at home services. If you are worried that by raising the issue of a will your relative will think you are after their money, there is a simple reply to this: you do not need to know what is in the will, you just need to ensure they have made one, so that in the event of their death, their estate can be divided as they would wish it to be. Anyone and everyone should make a will once they are self-sufficient and have income and/

or property, yet 30 per cent of over-50s in the UK have still not done so (see more on pages 27–32).

A Lasting Power of Attorney (LPA) allows you to take decisions on your loved one's behalf if they no longer have the mental capacity to do so. Many people have heard of a Lasting Power of Attorney (previously known as an Enduring Power of Attorney), but wrongly believe it is something to be considered only when mental incapacity sets in. If your relative suffers an accident or illness, you have no automatic right to act on their behalf. Without an existing LPA in place, you will be required to apply to the Court of Protection to be appointed as their deputy – a long, complex, costly and intrusive process. A relative cannot simply add their spouse or children to their bank accounts, as banks are instructed by the British Bankers' Association (BBA) to freeze both solely and jointly held accounts when one account holder loses mental capacity. If anything happens to your relative and a decision needs to be made about life-sustaining treatment, you can only do so if you have an LPA.

There are two types of LPA: property and financial, which deals with assets and financial affairs and health and welfare, which deals with medical and care issues. Your relative should grant both. It costs nothing to draw up a Lasting Power of Attorney, unless you want a solicitor's help to guide you through the correct process, which can be easier and more helpful than drafting it alone. It does, however, cost money to register an LPA. The forms you need are available to download from www.gov.uk.

An Advance Decision is a statement explaining what medical treatment the individual would not wish to have in the future, should that individual 'lack capacity', as defined by the Mental Capacity Act 2005. This statement does not have to be written down, although most are recorded as a written document as this is less likely to be challenged and will be valid in court if a dispute gets that far. Ideally, everyone should make an Advance Decision. This is because all of us are at risk of suddenly losing our capacity to make medical decisions for ourselves, if, for example, we become unconscious due to a car accident, a fall, or a stroke. Advance Decisions offer the opportunity to say what you do and do not want if that were to happen and take a great deal of pressure off your loved ones. Disputes about what is in an incapacitated person's best interests are often the subject of protracted court proceedings and so having an Advance Decision would avoid this problem. Read more detail on pages 40–42.

Essential care planning for older people

The first step is to think what your ideal care scenario would be and then talk to a specialist independent 'later life' financial advisor (not just a standard financial advisor). They will assess each individual situation thoroughly and advise on all conceivable options, including whether any state funding is available. Specialist later life financial planners will be authorised and regulated by the Financial Conduct Authority, and will also have obtained a dedicated long-term care qualification. They will be Disclosure and Barring Service checked too to provide added reassurance that they are cleared to provide guidance to vulnerable people. The Society of Later Life Advisers (SOLLA) is a good place to look for further information: www.societyoflaterlifeadvisers.co.uk.

Care fees have to be paid by the individual if their combined assets in terms of capital and property total more than £23,250, which is not very much at all. Hence, most people will have to fund all or part of their care and, therefore, it is essential to plan your relative's finances accordingly. There are certain allowances, however, which can be claimed based on a care assessment, such as attendance allowance, which is available to anyone over 65 who needs assistance with essential daily tasks for longer than six months. There are some scenarios where the NHS may be responsible for funding. If full-time care is required and a person's primary need is a health need, all their care fees could be paid by the NHS through NHS Continuing Health Care, although this is difficult to obtain.

Emergency contacts

It is a good idea to keep a list of the essential contacts relating to your relative in case of emergency. You can use the following chart as a guide to fill in and keep all the numbers you might need. You can also leave your relative with a copy by the phone. If your relative is comfortable using a mobile phone, you can also add an in case of emergency contact number. Keep it simple such as a name, i.e. Emergency or SOS.

Emergency telephone numbers for carers to complete and keep

Contact	*Tel No*	*Mobile No*	*Speed Dial Number*
Doctor's surgery			
Doctor Out of Hours			
Dentist			
Emergency dentist			
Local hospital			
Social worker			
Care worker			
Plumber			
Electrician			
Electricity supplier			
Water supplier			
Gas supplier			
Neighbour 1			
Neighbour 2			
Family/friend 1			
Family/friend 2			
Family/friend 3			
Local authority			

You can also create a shorter version for your relative to keep in their purse or wallet when they are out and about, in case of problems.

Emergency card for your relative to carry

	Your Details	*Emergency Contact Details 1*	*Emergency Contact Details 2*
Name D.O.B NHS No Dr: Name Dr: Tel Allergies			

CHAPTER FOUR

Essential Legal Decisions

Why it is imperative to make a will

Fifty-five per cent of adults aged under 55 and 35 per cent of those over 55 in the UK have not yet made a will. Many of us don't like to think about our own mortality, or we assume that our partner will inherit everything, should we die. This is not always the case, however, and siblings and relatives can also have a claim on your property unless you specify your exact wishes in a will. For instance, living as 'man and wife' does not mean that the law regards you as such. If one partner owns the property that two are living in, then the next of kin might be able to force a sale of the property, despite the other partner still living in it. If you die intestate (without a will), your spouse or civil partner will only receive a certain amount of your estate (currently the first £250,000, plus half of everything above that amount). They may also inherit if you have informally separated, but not if you have divorced or legally ended your civil partnership. Intestacy is the condition of the estate of a person who dies without having made a valid will or other binding declaration.

So it is very important to make a will to ensure that the intended beneficiaries from your estate receive their entitlement when you die. These could be relatives, friends or charities. The creation of a will leaves no uncertainty or ambiguity and eliminates disputes arising in the absence of a will. Working out the spouse's entitlement without a will may be very complex and extremely costly. If there is no spouse or children, the estate will go to more distant relatives, with whom you may have had no contact with for years, while close friends are excluded.

What happens if someone does not make a will?

Dying without a will means that you die intestate. Where there is no will, in an ideal scenario, the family would share the deceased's estate equally and amicably. This requires every family member to work unselfishly as a collective. As you can imagine, this can often lead to acrimony, especially if there are large amounts of money involved. When dividing the estate of someone who dies without a will, the rules of intestacy apply, which are that the spouse will receive all personal items and the first £250,000. In addition, they will receive a life interest in half the remainder of the estate. The rest of the estate will go to children, or even other distant relatives, and this could result in Inheritance Tax being paid. (Further information below on pages 32–35)

The case of Bob Marley is one of the most famous examples of what happens when someone does not make a will. The reggae star died of cancer at the age of 36, leaving a legacy of millions, but no will. After his death, his widow and mother fell out acrimoniously and the court-appointed administrator of the state tried to evict his mother from a house Marley had given to her. The Marley family are still arguing about his estate, nearly 40 years after his death.

What should you consider when making a will?

There is a raft of important questions to consider when making a will. You need to decide who you would like to choose as your executors, i.e. the people who would administer the estate when you die. You must choose someone you trust absolutely, who knows you well and who is a good administrator. If there are children under 18 years, you must make decisions on guardianship and specify this within the will. In a will, you can also leave legacies to relatives, friends and charities. It is important to note that any gift you leave to a charity is exempt from Inheritance Tax (IHT). As regards the residue, which is everything that is left after payment of debts, funeral expenses and IHT, you must decide who will receive those monies and in what proportions they will be paid.

You can write your own will, but there is more chance of getting it wrong legally and leaving it open to misinterpretation. If there are errors, the will may be considered invalid and then intestacy rules will apply. It is not recommended to write your own will unless the estate is very small and consists only of money and not of property. If the will is unclear, or it is not signed properly, then it could be declared invalid. Will writers are a cheaper alternative to solicitors, but unlike solicitors, they do not have to be qualified or regulated. They tend to be cheaper, but will not be able to advise on tax planning and Inheritance Tax matters. Solicitors can be more expensive, but they are more expert than lower-cost DIY services. Often they offer fixed fees for drafting a will, so ask for a fixed quote. The charges for drawing up a will vary between solicitors and also depend on the complexity of the will. Before making a decision on who to use, it is always advisable to check with a few local solicitors to find out how much they charge. You may have access to legal advice through an addition to an insurance policy, which might cover the costs of a solicitor preparing or checking a will, so it is worth checking your policies. If you are a member of a trade union, you may find that the union offers a free wills service to members and many companies also offer will writing as a staff benefit.

To save time and reduce costs when going to a solicitor, you should give some thought to the major points which you want included in your will. You should consider such things as:

- How much money and what property and possessions you have; for example, property, savings, occupational and personal pensions, insurance policies, bank and building society accounts, shares
- Who you want to benefit from your will. You should make a list of all the people to whom you wish to leave money or possessions. These people are known as beneficiaries. You also need to consider whether you wish to leave any money to charity

- Who should look after any children under 18. It is very important to ask the people you wish to name as guardian to accept this possible role prior to naming them on your will
- Who is going to sort out the estate and carry out your wishes as set out in the will. These people are known as the executors. Choose an executor whom you trust to be impartial and effective. Ideally choose a person or people who you believe will outlive you
- Once a will has been made, it should be kept in a safe place, either at home, with your solicitor or accountant, or at a bank.

Digital wills

Managing people's affairs after death is now more complicated with the advent of digital technology. Estates are normally left in a normal written will, a legal document which allows a person to give instructions on what to do with their possessions once they pass away and to declare a legal guardian for their children. However, now you also need to consider what happens to your digital assets and online presence when the inevitable happens. You need to ensure that someone else could access all your accounts for business and personal use. A digital will allows you to manage your online presence and assets in one document, without having to make arrangements with each site individually, as not all sites allow you to do this. Your website names, website addresses, usernames, passwords and any other relevant information, such as security questions and answers, will be stored in one place, ensuring your family has everything they need when the time comes.

How do you make a digital will?

You will need to write your digital will and assign your digital assets to your friends and family. Once your death is certified, your digital assets will be sent to those whom you have pre-chosen, be that family, friends or a solicitor. There are companies which allow you to manage all your passwords and online information in one, secure place, so it is worth searching online to find these. With some, you can also store notes for other types of important information, make your last wishes known and even attach documents, photos and leave messages for your loved ones. There are, however, a few obstacles to bear in mind:

- Make sure you include all the information needed and that all passwords are listed. Without them, online accounts cannot be accessed
- When using an online site to create your will, make sure it uses encryption, which converts information or data into a code. This will keep your online will safe and secure
- Be sure it is noted if any accounts need two-factor authentication, which is an extra layer of security used to ensure that people trying to gain access to an online account are who they say they are. First, a user will enter their username and a password. Then, instead of immediately gaining access, they will be required to provide another piece of information. This can be sent as a text to your phone, or might possibly be a code or password you have pre-agreed
- Make sure you provide any further detail needed to allow beneficiaries to log in, such as reminders for passwords, etc
- Remember that in order to access the information in the digital will, your family members will need to show proof of a death certificate to online networks and digital executors
- Digital wills may also go against the terms of service agreements of many websites. For instance, if it says in their terms that they cancel on death, you may not be able to transfer accounts to another individual
- Some websites, such as Google, Facebook and Instagram, provide the ability to activate a digital heir, so check and set this up if the service is available
- Within Google, there is an inactive account manager feature, which allows you to pick up to 10 trusted contacts, who will be notified if your account goes inactive and will be given access to your data (with your permission)
- Facebook and Instagram allow you to select someone so they can memorialise your page.

Never include your passwords or other digital asset access information in your Last Will and Testament. Your will becomes a public document once you have passed away, so anyone can read the sensitive information it may contain. In the will, just refer to an outside document which contains all the necessary information needed to settle your digital estate. Then you will be able to maintain your digital will, update it and add to it without having to change your will formally, or put your digital assets at risk. And remember, in the UK, only a Last Will and Testament on paper, signed in ink by appropriate witnesses, will be legally recognised. Although your 'digital will' could contain information about where your Last Will and Testament can be found, it cannot be used instead of a Last Will and Testament and a digital will may not stand up in a court of law.

Changing your will

After you have made a will, you can make a major change by signing a new will in the future if circumstances alter. A new will revokes any past will already made. After death, a will can be amended by a *deed of variation* by your executors and beneficiaries within two years of your passing. Also known as a deed of family arrangement, a deed of variation allows beneficiaries to rearrange or vary their entitlement. A deed of variation can be used by any person who receives a gift under a will to redirect their inheritance to another person. This person can be chosen irrespective of whether or not they are named in the will. Changes can be made only if all the beneficiaries agree.

Changing a will by deed of variation is very complex, so it is essential that you seek independent legal advice in any such matter.

What is Inheritance Tax (IHT)?

Inheritance Tax is a tax levied on the estate of someone who has died. Your estate includes all property, money and personal possessions.

You do not have to pay Inheritance Tax if the value of your estate falls below the current threshold of £325,000, or if you leave everything above that threshold to your spouse, or civil partner, or indeed to a charity. Tax rates change, so check for the most current threshold allowance on www.gov.uk. Even if the value of the estate of the deceased falls below the threshold, you must still report the value to HMRC.

If the deceased has gifted their home to their children, which can include stepchildren, adopted children and foster children, the threshold can increase to £450,000.

If you are married or in a civil partnership with an estate worth less than £325,000, any unused threshold should be added to your partner's threshold when you die, so that ultimately, their threshold could be as high as £900,000.

The standard Inheritance Tax rate is 40 per cent. This tax rate is only charged on the value of the estate above the threshold of £325,000. So if your estate is worth £750,000, you will only pay 40 per cent tax on £425,000, i.e. £750,000 minus the threshold of £325,000 = £425,00. At 40 per cent, the tax payable would be £170,000 in total. Note that if you leave more than 10 per cent or more of the net value of your estate to charity, the current 40 per cent tax due on the amount above the current threshold reduces to 36 per cent. As mentioned above, tax rates do change, so check for the latest rates at www.gov.uk.

Inheritance Tax and your home

Inheritance Tax is paid out of the estate by the person dealing with the deceased's wishes as expressed in the will. This person is called the executor. See pages 27–33 for further details on wills. Beneficiaries, i.e. the people who are given things in the will, do not usually have to pay tax on things they inherit, but there may be related taxes, such as costs associated with any property left to them in the will if they choose to rent it out. People may also have to pay tax on gifts given to them by the deceased, if that person dies within seven years of making that gift and has given away more than the £325,000 threshold. See below for more detail on what is allowed when gifting.

You are allowed to pass on your own home to your spouse or civil partner when you die and in this case, they will not pay Inheritance Tax. However, if you leave your home to someone other than a spouse or civil partner in your will, it will be valued as part of the estate. If you own your home, your tax-free threshold may increase to £450,000 if you leave the house to your children, or your estate value is less than £2,000,000.

Please note that if you want to carry on living in your home after giving it away, you will have to pay rent to the new owner at a suitable rate, i.e. the going rate for the area and not a nominal fee. In addition, you will also have to pay your share of the bills and continue to live there for another seven years. However, if you only give away part of the home *and* the new owners live with you, you do not have to pay rent.

If you die within seven years of giving away all or part of your property, your home will be treated as a gift. The seven-year rule will apply and the home will be liable for Inheritance Tax as outlined above.

Inheritance Tax and gifts

You do not have to pay Inheritance Tax on small gifts – for example, Christmas or birthday presents. You can gift as much as you like to your spouse or civil partner during your lifetime, as long as they live in the UK permanently.

To anyone other than your spouse or civil partner, you can make up to £3,000 worth of gifts each tax year, which will not be included in the value of your estate. You can also gift wedding or civil ceremony gifts to the value of £1,000 per person, as well as £2,500 for each grandchild or great-grandchild and £5,000 for each child. You can also make payments to help someone else to pay their living costs, such as an older relative or person under the age of 18. Gifts to charities and political parties are also exempt from Inheritance Tax.

Inheritance Tax on gifts outside the criteria outlined above is charged at 40 per cent on those gifts given in the three years before death. Gifts made three to seven years before are taxed on a sliding scale. This is called taper relief.

Taper relief:

Years between gift and death	*Tax paid*
Less than 3	40%
3 to 4	32%
4 to 5	24%
5 to 6	16%
6 to 7	8%
7 or more	0%

Clare died on 30 September, 2017. She did not have a spouse or civil partner. Six and a half years before she died, she gifted £300,000 to her sister, Suzanne. Four and a half years before she died, she gave £50,000 to her brother, Bruce, and she gave a friend, Caroline, £150,000 three and a half years before she died.

Clare had the £325,000 inheritance tax allowance, but nearly all of that was used up by her gift to her sister, Suzanne. There was no tax due on the gift to her sister as it was under the threshold. The remaining £25,000 of Clare's allowance went towards the gift she made to Bruce, but there was now tax to pay on the other £25,000 of that gift, payable at 24 per cent, in line with taper relief. The £150,000 Clare gave to Suzanne, her friend, was taxed at 32 per cent according to taper relief.

The rest of Clare's estate was worth £500,000, and that was taxable at 40 per cent.

If the deceased person lived abroad, Inheritance Tax would only be payable on any UK assets they might hold. HMRC will consider that the deceased lived in the UK if they lived in the UK for 15 of the past 20 years, or if they lived in the UK at any time during the last three years of their life.

Agreeing power of attorney (LPA)

If someone is anticipating health difficulties which mean they might not be able to make their own decisions anymore, they may need help managing their finances and/or their health issues. A Lasting Power of Attorney (LPA) is a legal document, where someone (while they still have mental capacity as certified by a solicitor) nominates a trusted friend or relative to look after their affairs if they lose capacity. It is essential to note that power of attorney cannot be granted once the person in question no longer has capacity, so this must be arranged before they become too ill or incapacitated.

There are two types of Lasting Power of Attorney.

1) The Property and Financial Affairs Lasting Power of Attorney enables people to deal with someone's finances – for example, to invest money on their behalf, pay bills and even sell their property.
2) The Health and Welfare Lasting Power of Attorney enables people to make decisions on someone's behalf about where they live, who looks after them and their ongoing medical care. They can also give their attorney power to make decisions about life-sustaining treatment.

What happens if your relative does not create a Lasting Power of Attorney (LPA)?

If an LPA has not been made and that authority has not been given, the only alternative for you to be able to manage their affairs on their behalf is to apply to the Court of Protection for the appointment of a person called a deputy. A deputy is a person appointed by the Court of Protection to manage the affairs and make decisions on behalf of the incapacitated person. The key reason to avoid this is the fact that it is genuinely so much easier to deal with someone's affairs who has put Lasting Power of Attorney in place rather than not. Dealing with a deputy is expensive and can be extremely time-consuming. Unless it is urgent, it can take six months to appoint a deputy successfully, and if a law firm is instructed, it is then necessary to deal with additional legal costs and court fees as well. Not only is the deputy responsible for the day-to-day management of the person's financial affairs, but he or she must be aware of, and respond to, essential issues at different stages of the patient's life. So, not having an LPA means things are far more complicated.

Importantly, someone can only set up a Lasting Power of Attorney when they have mental capacity. Once you have lost capacity, it is simply too late. In order to set this up, a solicitor must interview the person wanting to create an LPA in order to assess whether they still have the mental capacity to decide. In addition, the process of making an LPA can help prompt broader discussions with your relative's family or others about his or her future wishes. It is always better to have these discussions within a calm environment when everyone involved has the time to focus.

For all these reasons, it makes perfect sense for everyone to make a Lasting Power of Attorney before they become too incapacitated to do so. Setting up each LPA currently costs £82, so £164 for both, which can make it difficult to afford for some people, but it is very much worth the outlay if you can find the money and it may well save you money in the long run.

It is also worth considering taking out Lasting Power of Attorney between spouses or partners in case either one of you should become suddenly incapacitated much earlier in life, which can happen due to sudden illness or accident.

Dorothy refused to register for an LPA. When she finally had to go into a care home and was no longer able to make decisions for herself, the local authority took charge of her affairs and her family was unable to direct the decisions on her behalf. Eventually, they were granted the power to act on her behalf by the Court of Protection, but by then, Dorothy was very frail and died shortly afterwards. Her daughter, Pat, commented, 'It was distressing enough having to put Mum into a home, but having no say over her legal, financial or care decisions was a nightmare, as was the process of going through the courts. Whatever you do, get the LPAs sorted before you get to the position we found ourselves in. We were essentially powerless to help her.'

How can you persuade your relative to set up an LPA?

One of the difficulties with creating LPAs can be resistance from your relative. This is understandable, as people do not want to have discussions about what happens if they lose their faculties, or when they are going to die. If you are going to conduct those discussions with your relative, you may want to consider what you will say and how you will say it and when. Preparation with a positive outcome in mind is essential to enable them to provide the necessary consent willingly. Try to project reassurance as many older people (or indeed anyone) can be concerned about discussing something of which they are afraid, namely their loss of faculties and their independence. You must be sympathetic in recognising this potential distress, by pointing out that this is something that everyone might eventually need, and in fact that you may already have with your own partner. Listen to any objections quietly, try to understand where they are coming from and do not rise to any provocation. Dealing with family issues is potentially difficult for all of us. If your relative is very difficult when you discuss this issue, do your best to maintain composure. Remaining calm and discussing the benefits rationally usually convinces people in the end. Just keep returning to the subject at the right times.

If you are not comfortable having those discussions yourself, consider using a trusted friend or advisor to talk with your relative. You may wish to consider using a solicitor with good negotiation skills, who is independent and has the credibility to address any objections in a rational manner. Ideally, he or she can bring a family with differing interests and views together. Given the stress which family members can suffer when arranging legal and financial issues for their relatives, the trusted advisor may be the best way to go, in order to minimise the prospect of conflict in these difficult times.

Remember, registering an LPA does not give you the automatic right to take over your relative's affairs on completion of registration. An LPA can only be triggered once you have applied to the solicitor and obtained a doctor's authorisation that the LPAs should now be implemented due to incapacity. Only then can you act as their attorney.

Registration of an LPA

In England, Wales and Scotland, you have to register an LPA before you can use it. In Northern Ireland, you can use it without registering while your relative still has mental capacity, but you have to register it as soon as their mental capacity starts to decline. In either case, it is best to register as soon as possible. This is because during the registration process, the document will be checked for errors. If you catch them while your relative can still manage their affairs, you can correct them. If not, your Lasting Power of Attorney might be invalid.

Current fees for England and Wales are £82 for each Lasting Power of Attorney. In Northern Ireland, it costs £115 for each Enduring Power of Attorney and in Scotland, it is £75 for each Power registered. The fees may change, so it is a good idea to check when you register on www.gov.uk. However, if you paid to register a Lasting Power of Attorney in England or Wales between 1 April, 2013 and 31 March, 2017, you are owed a refund of up to £54. Under a new government scheme announced in February 2018, those who paid a registration fee for a Lasting Power of Attorney during that period can apply for a partial refund as they were charged more than was necessary. From 2013, the Office of the Public Guardian's operating costs went down, but the application fee stayed the same, so the government is now repaying some of the cash. You can claim via the Court of Protection.

If you decide to cancel an LPA, you can draw up a deed of revocation. In order to do this, you need to send the Office of the Public Guardian

(OPG) both the original LPA and a written statement called a deed of revocation. This should read:

'This deed of revocation is made by [your name] of [your address].

1: I granted a lasting power of attorney for property and financial affairs/health and welfare (delete as appropriate) on [date you signed the Lasting Power of Attorney] appointing [name of first attorney] of [address of first attorney] and [name of second attorney] of [address of second attorney] to act as my attorney(s).

2: I revoke the Lasting Power of Attorney and the authority granted by it.

Signed and delivered as a deed [your signature]

Date signed [date]

Witnessed by [signature of witness]

Full name of witness [name of witness]

Address of witness [address of witness]

You can find all the forms you need online at www.gov.uk.

Making an Advance Decision/Living Will

Ideally, everyone should make an advance decision. This is because all of us are at risk of suddenly losing our capacity to make medical decisions for ourselves, such as if we become unconscious due to a car accident, a fall, or a stroke, for example. Some of us sadly already know that we are going to lose capacity sooner rather than later, in particular, people with a progressive neurological disease, or perhaps mild memory loss, which might render the person at risk of progressing to dementia. Advance decisions offer the opportunity to say what you do and do not want if that were to happen.

At a time when person-centred care and the rights and dignity of the individual are paramount, advance decisions are featuring more and more in the legal and medical landscape. They are important documents both to safeguard and promote an individual's health and interests. Crucially, they allow someone to maintain their dignity.

If, for example, an individual was in medical need of treatment (such as a blood transfusion, an amputation, or a feeding tube) and was unable to make their own decision at the time (e.g. because they were unconscious), the advance decision would tell doctors if the person had refused such treatment.

Disputes about what is in an incapacitated person's best interests are often the subject of protracted court proceedings, which can be costly and distressing, and having an advance decision would avoid this.

A woman in a minimally conscious state was refused an application to withdraw artificial nutrition and hydration, allowing her to die. Without engaging in ethical and moral discussions about the rights and wrongs inherent in this judgment, if the woman had had an advance decision specifying, 'I refuse artificial nutrition and hydration if I am ever in a minimally conscious state', (which is what her family believed that she would have said), then that would have been legally binding.

How to ensure an Advance Decision is legally binding

To ensure your advance decision is legally binding, you must be over the age of 18 and have capacity to understand information relevant to the decision, to remember that information and to weigh up the pros and cons of your decisions. Unless you have an impairment or disorder of the mind or brain (a mental illness, brain injury or dementia), this is assumed to be the case. Even if you do have an impairment, it is often possible for you to make an advance decision with appropriate support, as long as you have stated the specific treatments you want to refuse and clearly listed the set of circumstances in which treatment would be refused, stating, '*I maintain these refusals even if my life is shortened as a result*'. You must also ensure that it is properly witnessed. This can be done by the GP.

It is important to review your advance decision if there are particular changes in your circumstances (e.g. if you have a new diagnosis), but the assumption otherwise is that the advance decision is valid unless or until you revoke it. If you have an old living will, or an advance decision that is more than two or three years old, however, it would be a good idea to review it, make any changes you want, and sign it and get it witnessed again. Make sure that your family and your GP are aware of your advance decision.

How to manage the probate process

When someone dies, the executors (those people nominated by the deceased to manage their will) need to apply for a grant of probate, which allows them access to the property and possessions within the estate. If someone dies with a will, they will be granted probate, but if they die intestate (without a will), they will not. For more details on wills, see pages 27–32. You may not need to apply for probate if the deceased owned land, property, shares on money jointly, or if they only had savings or premium bonds.

When you apply for probate, you need to value the deceased person's estate (i.e. the money, property and possessions). To do this, you must establish their assets and debts. You will need to contact banks, pension companies, investment companies etc. as relevant and utilities, such as gas, electricity and phone companies. You will also need to get the property valued by a reputable estate agent. The value of the estate will determine if and how much Inheritance Tax you will have to pay. This will be decided by HMRC once you have submitted all the details needed to apply for a grant of probate. It can take from a couple of months to well over a year to gain probate, depending on the complexity of the estate.

If someone dies intestate (without a will), you can ask to be an administrator of the estate. Usually this is next of kin, i.e. a spouse, civil partner, or child. Once you have applied to be an administrator, you will receive letters of administration certifying you to deal with the estate. You will then follow the probate process as outlined above. However, if the deceased died intestate, the law decides who inherits the estate. See pages 27–28 for more details on intestacy.

It is essential to get good legal advice when dealing with probate or letters of administration. Beware companies charging high fees for probate. Some specialist probate companies can charge exorbitant prices for the service, far more than solicitors. These companies may be recommended by funeral providers, or may even be printed on documents with the death certificate, so beware. Some probate specialists and solicitors charge an hourly rate, while others charge a fee that is a percentage of the value of the estate. This fee is usually calculated as between 1 to 5 per cent of the value of the estate, plus VAT.

The table below is an example of how much you could end up paying for probate services. This total doesn't include court or application fees, so the final bill is probably higher.

Value of estate	*Fees*	*VAT*	*Total payable*
£100,000	£1,000 (1% of estate value)	£200	£1,200
£100,000	£5,000 (5% of estate value)	£1,000	£6,000

Some probate specialists charge both an hourly rate and a percentage fee, but this doesn't necessarily mean they are more expensive. There are also a few probate specialist companies who charge a fixed fee for their services. They base it on an estimate of the volume of work involved. These companies claim to be cheaper than a traditional solicitor or accountant.

Most banks also offer probate and estate administration services. However, these services are often more expensive than using a solicitor or a specialist company.

If you are concerned about the cost, you can get more than one quote for probate.

When Anthony had to administer his late mother's estate, it took over three years. The firm he used ran up significant costs, way over what he had expected, although he never obtained a definitive quotation initially, just an estimate. When challenged, the solicitors claimed it was due to a change in personnel and 'additional advice', without giving any further clarification. When Anthony complained and asked for some indication of the final bill, he was told that it would be over double the sum originally estimated. He had no choice but to pay it in order to settle the probate proceedings.

CHAPTER FIVE

Financial Planning

Trying to make sensible decisions about how to fund care is very difficult, especially when you are dealing with an emotional family situation. There are so many things to think about, such as the type of care your relative might need, what their own wishes are and how to agree to a solution that works for your relative. You want to keep your relative as happy as possible, while ensuring that the care solution also works for you.

The question of how to fund care is often the last consideration, but care is very expensive and we should all be planning for how to pay for it well before we reach old age. Most of us plan for retirement and how we intend to pay for care should be an essential part of that planning process. It used to be the case that most people only needed care for two or three years at the end of their life, but as life expectancy continues to increase, this can often now extend beyond 10 years.

Care is means tested. Those people who have assets above the current means test threshold of £23,250, and do not qualify for NHS Continuing Care, have to pay for their own care. NHS Continuing Care is when the NHS agrees to fund all care costs and it is very difficult to obtain. £23,250 includes all assets, including a person's total capital and their home. Hence, it is very important to plan ahead to pay for care as the majority of people in the UK do not qualify for NHS Continuing Care. You can find out more on pages 59–62.

Beware: Do not be tempted to encourage your relative to put their home in your name to reduce their assets. If this has been done in close proximity to requesting NHS Continuing Care, it will not be allowed to stand. The only way to do this is for your relative to gift their home to you more than seven years ahead of requiring care (see pages 32–35 on Inheritance Tax and gifting for more detail). Gifting a home in itself can be open to unscrupulous practices by some families, who then use the home as their asset and the older person may lose out.

When looking at finances in later life, start by collating all financial information, including bank statements, savings and investment statements, details of state pension and any other benefits, such as attendance allowance, which provides money for care services at home (see pages 54–56 for more details). Check that all benefits are being claimed, as often people are entitled to benefits, but have not claimed for them. Add up all the income and consider any expenses that will continue to be paid, in addition to the care home fees. This may include household costs if the home is being kept, or while it is being sold. Also consider any personal expenses that may be incurred in the care home, such as hairdressing and shopping for personal items and clothing. Then consider the difference between income and expenditure and this will give you the shortfall that has to be covered from your relative's assets.

If there is a property involved, consider whether you wish this to be sold or rented out. It is sensible to take advice from a few estate agents on any remedial work needed and if selling, decide what price will achieve a quick sale (if this is what is required), or if renting, decide what is a suitable level of rent. Bear in mind that, if renting, there may be periods with no tenant and it may be necessary to spend capital on repairs, etc. It is a good idea to take advice on all options from an independent financial adviser who specialises in later life issues.

There are three main options to find capital to help meet the shortfall in care costs. All have advantages and disadvantages, and no one route is the perfect answer for everyone.

The first is to place all capital on deposit, either in an instant access account, or by using fixed term accounts as appropriate. This is the simplest option to understand and operate as funds can be transferred quickly and accessed easily to pay for care costs and other expenses, depending on the accounts used. However, current poor interest rates mean that capital can run down very quickly and for large sums, it may be difficult to administer if you are trying to keep bank balances below the Financial Services Compensation Scheme limit of £85,000. This scheme offers reimbursement up to £85,000 in one bank should the bank collapse, but will not protect amounts over £85,000.

Secondly, you can consider stock market-related investments to fund care, such as unit trusts or other funds, which involves placing a reserve amount of capital (say 12 months' expenses) into a deposit account and investing the remainder with a view to receiving more income than you would by placing the money in a deposit account. This provides the potential for higher income than placing the money in deposit accounts and yields possibly greater capital growth, but you must bear in mind that investment values can fall as well as rise and as a result, the benefits of extra income can be outweighed by falls in capital value. A good understanding of the risks involved with investments is necessary and therefore you should always seek advice from an independent financial adviser.

Finally, care annuities allow you to pay an amount of capital to an insurance company in return for a guaranteed pre-agreed income to a care provider for the rest of your relative's life. This is calculated after an assessment of an individual's own specific circumstances and health. Annuities can provide a high and increasing income, paid tax-free direct to a registered care provider for life, however long that may be, and can protect at least some of the available capital.

They can also provide peace of mind that capital will never run out. Annuities continue to be paid even if your older relative qualifies for NHS Continuing Care funding, or is returning home, although a small amount of tax is then payable on each income payment. However, a large capital outlay at the outset means that care annuities can be poor value if death occurs in the early years. Annuities are also inflexible, as once purchased, it is not possible to change the terms if circumstances change. Income payments are fixed (or increase at a pre-agreed rate) and therefore, this may not be a suitable option if care needs are likely to increase in the future, e.g. a move from residential to nursing or dementia care.

These are just some of the options available and in some cases a mixture of approaches is appropriate. It is very important that qualified and experienced specialist financial advice is sought at as early a stage as possible to ensure an informed decision is taken. Suitable local advisers can be found on the Society of Later Life Advisers (SOLLA) website, www.societyoflaterlifeadvisers.co.uk, or you can get further advice on this subject from Age UK www.ageuk.org.uk, or from Citizens Advice www.citizensadvice.org.uk.

Direct payments and personal budgets for care at home

Following assessment of an older person's requirements, the local authority can charge for the services it arranges for an older person at home, dependent on means testing. Only the person receiving the services will be financially assessed. The assessors will ask questions about the person's financial circumstances to see how much, if anything, they can contribute towards the cost of services.

The procedures for charging for care in a person's own home and the amounts charged vary between local authorities, but charges should always be 'reasonable'. Government guidance sets out a broad framework for the local authority to follow, so an older person should be able to afford to receive services and not be pushed into poverty.

The local authority will calculate the cost of the services to be provided (such as home care, meals, transport, etc.) and then financially assess the person using their own charging policy, to see how much they can contribute to the cost of the services. The local authority must provide a breakdown of how they worked out the charge.

Direct payments

Rather than receive services arranged by the local authority, the person, or their carer, may choose to be given a direct payment from the local authority so they can arrange relevant care services for themselves. The local authority must be satisfied that the person is willing and able to manage a direct payment, either alone, or with assistance. Direct payments may offer more choice and flexibility, but they can be complicated to handle and rules vary from area to area. The local authority must support that person managing a direct payment, which may be through voluntary or charitable services.

If the person lacks the mental capacity to consent to a direct payment, a 'suitable person' can act as an agent and receive and manage the direct payment on their behalf. The suitable person may be an attorney designated under a registered Power of Attorney, a court-appointed deputy, carer, or a relative or friend. The local authority must be satisfied that the suitable person will act in the best interests of the person, especially if they have dementia.

If your local authority (or your Health and Social Care Trust in Northern Ireland) agrees to fund some or all of your relative's care services, you will be offered the choice of the council providing the services directly to your relative, or receiving direct payments from the council, and arranging and paying for the care and support services yourself. To receive direct payments, first you need to contact your relative's local council or trust to ask them to assess their care needs. How much they get depends on their financial circumstances and they may need to top it up with money of their own. Direct payments go straight into your relative's bank, building society, Post Office, or National Savings account, but they cannot just spend the money on anything – the council has to be satisfied that the money is buying services to help provide legitimate care needs, as agreed in your relative's care plan. If the local authority thinks that a direct payment has not been properly used, it can try to recover some, or all, of the payment. It could ask your relative to repay if either of the following apply:

- They have not used all or part of the direct payment to buy the services which the payment was intended to pay for
- The direct payment was made subject to a condition which has not been met.

If the local authority demands that your relative must repay a direct payment, you should get advice from Citizens Advice.

There have been numerous cases of fraud relating to direct payments, where family members or friends have redirected money for themselves, but beware. The local authorities are adept at investigating fraud successfully and perpetrators receive lengthy jail sentences.

Direct payments could be right for you and your relative if they want to retain or take control of their own care and support services, or if they want more choice in selecting the products and services that meet their specific needs. They are a good choice if you and your relative are confident with money and paperwork, or have people to support you with this and you are happy to keep receipts and invoices and submit these to social services on time. Also, do remember that if you employ carers directly with this budget, you are responsible for paying tax, National Insurance and pension for them as an employee. Or you can ask a care agency to supply you with managed care, which costs more, but the advantage is that they will handle tax, National Insurance and pensions on your behalf.

Personal budgets

A personal budget is an up-front allocation of funding to meet the person or carer's eligible needs. The allocation may be:

- retained by the local authority and 'earmarked' for the person's needs, or managed through an individual service fund, which is paid to a third party, such as a care agency
- managed through a user-controlled trust, which is run by trustees and spent on the person's behalf
- paid directly to the person, a carer or suitable person if the person lacks mental capacity.

If the person, or their carer, decides that they want the local authority to retain their personal budget, they should still be involved in deciding which services should be commissioned to best meet their needs.

Complaining about care

If the person being cared for, or their carer, has a complaint, it is advisable to try and sort it out with the person they have contact with, such as the assessor or care manager. There may simply have been a failure in communication, or a misunderstanding that can be easily rectified. However, if this is not successful, there is a local authority complaints procedure. The individual local authority will explain how to use this. The complaints procedure might be useful if there are problems arranging an assessment, if there is an unreasonably long wait for an assessment, or if the services needed are not provided, or are unsatisfactory. If the local authority complaints procedure does not resolve the issue either, you can take your complaint to the Local Government Ombudsman.

Claiming on insurance to cover care costs

Make sure you check to see if you can claim on any existing insurance policies to pay for care. Many people have taken out some kind of health insurance in the past, which might be helpful when it comes to paying for care. Check if your relative holds any of the following:

- life insurance with critical illness cover
- a standalone critical illness policy
- long-term care insurance policy – although these are no longer available, they were very popular at one time
- an over-50s plan
- terminal illness cover (this might have been included when your relative took out their mortgage)
- income protection cover
- cover taken out on their behalf by a current employer or someone they have worked for in the past
- cover that someone else in the family has taken out on their behalf, or a joint policy taken out with their spouse or partner that will cover your relative if they become ill.

In order to claim, find as much of the original paperwork relating to the insurance policy as you can. If the policy was bought through a broker, contact them first. They might be able to support you, or manage the claim on your behalf.

Benefits and savings – what benefits can you claim over 60?

Many older people in the UK are unaware that they are entitled to receive cash benefits from the government from the age of 60. More than a million low-income pensioners fail to collect their pension credits every year, and they may also be missing out on other benefits, such as attendance allowance (see pages 54–56) and social care support that could help them with health costs.

Changes to the pension age by the government mean that if you were born after 1950, you will not be able to claim your state pension until you reach your mid-60s and many people will have to work up to and maybe even beyond that point. However, there are still some benefits which are available from the age of 60, which can help with costs associated with maintaining health.

These benefits include free prescriptions and sight tests. People under 60 may be eligible for free prescriptions earlier in Wales, Scotland and Northern Ireland. Check with the relevant government websites. To obtain the free benefits, simply fill in the form on the back of the prescription and hand it to your pharmacist. You may need to show proof of age. Men and women will also receive an invitation to be screened for bowel cancer every two years. For a full list of health screenings available to men and women, see the medical matters section on pages 153–159.

Personal Independence Payment (PIP)

Personal Independence Payments (PIPs) have replaced the Disability Living Allowance, aimed at helping children and adults under 65 who require financial help for assistance with personal care. PIP is designed to help cover some of the extra costs associated with a long-term condition, disability, or severe visual impairment. If your relative is under the age of 64, they could get between £22.65 and £145.35 a week (check www.gov.uk as payment amounts are subject to change). The amount your relative gets depends on how their condition affects them, not on the condition itself. A health professional will assess your relative to work out the level of help they can get and the rate will be regularly reviewed to ensure they are getting the right support. PIPs are non-means tested, so they do not rely on the amount of capital or property your relative has.

Personal Independence Payment is made up of two components. The mobility component might be paid if your relative needs help getting about. The daily living component might be paid if they need help with carrying out everyday activities, such as washing and dressing. Each component can be paid at either a standard or enhanced rate. Depending on how their condition affects them, it is possible to get one component or both, and at either the standard or the enhanced rate. You can find more information at www.gov.uk.

Winter fuel payments

Keeping warm is vital for older people and these one-off payments are made each winter to those over 60. Your relative will qualify for the winter fuel payment if they were born on or before 5 January 1953 (this date changes every year, so it is a good idea to check on the www.gov.uk website) and they were living in the UK throughout a particular eligibility week – for example, in 2018, this week was 17–23 September. This eligibility week changes annually, so check on www.gov.uk. People already receiving benefits will automatically receive the winter fuel payment. Your relative can also make a claim via www.gov.uk, or by calling their helpline on 0800 731 0160.

Cold weather payment

People who receive certain benefits, such as pension credit, income support and universal credit, may be entitled to a further payment of £25 if local temperatures drop, or they are forecast to fall to zero degrees Celsius or below for seven consecutive days between 1 November and 31 March.

Heating schemes

People on a low income, who live in poorly insulated homes or without central heating, as well as those receiving pension credit, can apply for state assistance. Different heating schemes are in place around the UK. You can contact the Home Heat Helpline on 0800 336699.

What benefits can you claim over 65?

Attendance allowance

Attendance allowance is a benefit payable to people aged 65 or over, who have attention or supervision needs, but are neither in hospital, nor living in a residential care setting. Entitlement requires a level of disability which results in a need for frequent attention from another person, either because of difficulty with bodily functions (i.e. eating, drinking, washing, toileting, mobility, seeing, hearing, etc.), or because supervision is required in order to prevent substantial danger to the claimant, or others. The disability condition must be met continually for a period of six months. Claimants must also be ordinarily resident in Great Britain and present in Great Britain both at the time of the claim and for 26 of the preceding 52 weeks. Depending on the degree of disability, the benefit is potentially payable at one of two rates: a higher rate of £85.60 per week and a lower rate of £57.30 per week. (Rates do change, so check on www.gov.uk.) Higher rate attendance allowance is also available for those who are terminally ill. If someone is a permanent resident in a care home and their place is wholly or partly funded by a local authority entitlement, attendance allowance can be affected.

When your relative applies for attendance allowance, make sure they (or you, if you are assisting them) have the accompanying notes with them as they will assist you to fill in the form. These notes are available at www.nidirect.gov.uk. If possible, print the notes off as it is useful to be able to refer to them as you go along. The forms are also available in larger print and braille for those who are vision impaired. Ask the GP to support your relative's application.

Top tip: Speak to the relevant GP before completing the form and ask them to agree to speak to the Department for Work and Pensions (DWP) about the application if they are contacted. This will prevent unnecessary hold-ups later in the process. Provide ALL the information you can and give as much detail as you can in the form.

Specifically, when thinking about the assistance you or your relative might require, think about the worst days rather than the best days, so you do not underestimate the care they might need. The issues you consider should include:

- help with personal hygiene
- incontinence issues
- help with dressing and undressing
- preparing, carrying and eating food
- help with sorting and taking medicines
- help with mobility around the home, including using the stairs
- help with getting in and out of chairs and in and out of the bath.

Think about the type of aids and home adaptation which might help. In particular, you should try to assess the risk of falls. You can also ask for help with visual or aural impairment and dementia.

Make sure that you, or another family member, complete the section at the end of the form, which asks for someone else's view on the situation as this will help your relative to get a positive outcome. You can ask their GP to do this if you prefer. If you are helping your relative to fill out the form, make sure they sign it personally unless you have been granted Power of Attorney over them. The form must be posted, not emailed.

Annual flu jab

Everybody aged 65 and over in the UK is eligible for a free flu jab every winter. The jabs are available in GP surgeries and pharmacies between September and February each year.

Help for older people on low incomes

Pension credit (PC)

It is estimated that about 4 million older people are entitled to pension credit, yet only about two-thirds of those eligible are claiming it.

Pension credit (PC) is a two-part income-related benefit: the guarantee credit – which tops up weekly income to a guaranteed minimum level – and the savings credit – which helps people whose income is higher than the basic state pension.

Guarantee Credit tops up your weekly income to a guaranteed minimum level, which is £163 if you're single, or £248.80 if you're a couple.

Savings Credit is extra money if you've got some savings, or your income is higher than the basic State Pension. It's only available to people who reached State Pension age before 6 April, 2016. You could get up to £13.40 extra per week if you're single, or £14.99 if you're a couple. These amounts do change, so check at www.gov.uk.

Even if your relative is only eligible for a small amount of PC, it is still worth applying for. Everyone receiving the guarantee credit portion of PC is entitled to free dental treatment and prescriptions, vouchers towards glasses/contact lenses, wigs, fabric supports and help with travel costs to hospital appointments.

The NHS Low Income Scheme

People on low incomes and with savings of less than £16,000 (or £23,500 if living in a residential care home) may be entitled to help from the NHS with costs associated with NHS prescriptions, NHS dental check-ups and treatment, glasses and contact lenses and travel costs to receive NHS treatment (if under the care of a consultant). Anyone can apply as long as they don't have savings or investments over a certain limit. You can't get help if you or your partner (or both) have more than £16,000 in savings, investments or property (not including the place where you live), or £23,250 in savings, investments or property if you live permanently in a care home (£24,000 if you live in Wales).

If you are over 60, don't live with a partner and your only income is from a pension, you might be able to apply online. You don't need to apply if you're already entitled to full help with health costs. You will get help with full health costs if you receive a Pension Credit Guarantee. You're also entitled to full help if you are named on, or entitled to, an NHS tax credit exemption certificate.

Full details of the scheme can be found on the NHS website, www.nhs.uk. Application forms for the NHS Low Income Scheme can be found at GP surgeries, hospitals, opticians and dentists.

Council tax reduction

Your relative can now apply for council tax reduction if they pay council tax and are on a low income and claiming certain benefits. They can apply for a council tax reduction whether they own their home, or if they rent. See www.gov.uk for details.

Council tax exemptions

A full council tax bill is based on at least two adults living in a house or flat. It is possible to get 25 per cent off the bill if your relative counts as an adult for council tax purposes (i.e. is over the age of 18) and lives on their own. They will also get a discount if they live with people who do not count as adults for council tax. Live-in carers who look after someone who is not their partner, spouse or child are not included in a home's council tax.

Travel allowances

Depending on your relative's age and where they live in the UK, they could be entitled to free or discounted bus travel. In some regions of the UK, they could also get concessions on rail and other fares. The Disabled Persons Railcard also provides a discount, with a third off most fares for the cardholder and a companion. Disabled drivers can apply under the Blue Badge scheme for a pass enabling them to park in some restricted areas, such as on yellow lines. The government's Motability scheme allows disabled people to lease a new car, mobility scooter or powered wheelchair without needing to pay road tax. If your relative was born before 3 September, 1929 and is a British national, they can apply for a free 10-year passport. Some products, including expensive purchases such as mobility vehicles, can be purchased without paying VAT, or at a reduced VAT rate of 5 per cent, if the buyer is registered disabled. This is subject to approval from HMRC and proof of disability.

TV

Your relative is able to get a free TV licence from the age of 75 and can apply for a short-term licence if they are 74, valid until the end of the month before they turn 75.

War pension

If your relative's spouse or civil partner has died as a result of their service in Her Majesty's Armed Forces, or during a time of war, they may be entitled to a war widow's or widower's pension. To claim, contact the Service Personnel and Veterans Agency on 0808 1914 2 18.

NHS Continuing Care

NHS Continuing Care (also known as fully funded NHS Care) is care that is arranged and funded by the NHS free of charge outside of hospital. It is available for people who need ongoing healthcare and meet the prescribed eligibility criteria. NHS Continuing Care can be provided in a care home, hospice or the home of the person who needs care. If someone in a care home is eligible for NHS Continuing Care, this will cover all care home fees, including cost of accommodation, personal care and healthcare. If NHS Continuing Care is provided at home, it covers personal care and healthcare costs. It may also include support for carers. To be eligible for NHS Continuing Care, the person must be assessed as having a 'primary health need' and must have a complex medical condition and ongoing care needs. Not everyone with long-term condition or disability is eligible. The assessment for NHS Continuing Care is supposed to be person-centred, i.e. the person being assessed should be fully involved in the assessment process. Their views about their own needs and support should be taken into account and they should be kept fully informed about the process. Carers are also involved, where appropriate. A decision about eligibility should usually be made within 28 days of an assessment being carried out.

If your relative does qualify for NHS Continuing Care, their local authority will be responsible for their care assessment and providing relevant services. If your relative does not qualify for NHS Continuing Care, but is assessed as having care or nursing needs, they can still receive some care from the NHS. For someone in their own home, this could be part of a joint package of care, with some services coming from the NHS and some from social services. If your relative moves into a nursing home, the NHS may contribute towards nursing care costs. If they are eligible for local authority care, their finances will be assessed. Depending on their income and savings, they may need to pay towards their care costs.

Primary care trusts must carry out an assessment for NHS Continuing Care if it seems that someone may need it. For example, the assessment should be carried out if someone's physical or mental health worsens significantly, before someone is awarded NHS-funded nursing care, or when someone is discharged from hospital. You can also ask for an assessment for your relative by talking to a health or social care worker, or to the NHS continuing healthcare coordinator at your relative's primary care trust. You can find out the name of your local coordinator by asking your GP, or by contacting the local Patient Advice and Liaison Service, or by contacting your relative's Clinical Commissioning Group directly.

The initial assessment is a checklist, completed by a nurse, doctor, other healthcare professional or social worker. Your relative should be told what is happening and be asked for their consent. Depending on the outcome, they will be told that they are either not eligible for NHS Continuing Care, or if they are eligible, they will be referred for a full assessment. Being referred for a full assessment does not necessarily mean your relative will ultimately be eligible for NHS Continuing Care, however, as it merely leads onto the next stage of the process. Whatever the decision, the professional completing the checklist should provide written reasons for their decision and sign and date the checklist. Your relative should be given a copy of the completed checklist. You can download a blank copy of the NHS Continuing Care checklist from www.gov.uk.

When your relative has a full assessment for NHS Continuing Care, a multi-disciplinary team, made up of health and social care professionals already involved in their care, will assess their care needs. This team will use a 'decision support tool', which is a document used to record an individual's needs, in order to decide whether your relative is eligible. The assessment looks at behaviour, cognition (understanding), communication, psychological and emotional needs, mobility, continence, skin problems, breathing, medication and altered states of consciousness. Those carrying out the assessment should look at what help is needed, how complex the needs are and assess any risks that would exist if adequate care was not provided. For each of these issues, a decision is then made about the level of need, marked as either priority, severe, high, moderate or low. If your relative has at least one priority need, or severe needs in at least two areas, they should be eligible for NHS Continuing Care. Someone can also qualify if they have a severe need in one area, plus a number of high or moderate needs.

The assessment should consider your relative's and your own views, and you should be given a copy of the completed decision support tool document with clear reasons for the decision. If someone's condition is deteriorating fast, they should be assessed under the NHS Continuing Care fast track pathway so that an appropriate care package can be put in place as soon as possible. Government guidance says that care should be put in place within 48 hours of someone being found eligible under the fast track pathway. You can find out more at www.nhs.uk.

Phyllis was granted NHS Continuing Care because of the many and varied problems she suffered. She had advanced Parkinson's disease. She had also suffered three strokes and had Parkinson's dementia. In addition, she had heart disease and was unable to walk. Hence Phyllis was dependent for most things (dressing, washing, eating, drinking, turning in bed, etc.) and was physically and mentally frail. She was mostly immobile and had no strength and little coordination of her limbs. She only weighed about 6 stone in weight. She had difficulty speaking and swallowing; she was also doubly incontinent.

Phyllis needed to sleep in a bed with bedrails down each side and had to be hoisted out of a chair or a bed. She was at severe risk of pressure sores and tissue breakdown. She experienced some involuntary and jerky movements of her limbs, consistent with Parkinson's disease. She was excessively sleepy and her eyes were closed most of the time, even if she was awake.

Without regular physiotherapy, she would have experienced permanent, chronic and painful contracture of her joints, which would have resulted in her needing even more care. She could sometimes say a few words coherently and acknowledge what was being said to her. The degree to which she was aware of her environment varied from day to day.

Pensions

Pensions provide a regular income once a person reaches state pension age. The pension is based on National Insurance contributions and the amount your relative gets depends on how much they have paid in.

There are three main types of pension, which are the state pension, defined benefit pensions, and defined contribution pensions.

State Pensions

Most people receive some state pension, paid by the government. This is secure income, which grows by at least the rate of inflation annually. Your state pension entitlement builds via the National Insurance contributions you make while you are working. From April 2016, a new flat rate state pension was introduced. For the tax year 2018/2019, the full new state pension was £164.35 per week. Figures change annually, so check at www.gov.uk. However, your relative might be entitled to more, if they have built up entitlement to additional state pension based on the pre-April 2016 system – or maybe even less than this, if they contracted out of the additional state pension. To be eligible, your relative will usually need a minimum of 10 qualifying years on their National Insurance record.

If you are widowed, you might inherit an extra payment, as well as part of your deceased partner's additional state pension if you married or entered into a civil partnership prior to 6 April, 2016 and your partner reached state pension age before 6 April, 2016, or if they died before 6 April, 2016, but would have been of state pension age on or after that date.

Defined Benefit Pension

You would normally have a defined benefit (DB) pension if you have worked for a big company, or in the public sector. It is a salary-related pension, paying out a secure income for life, which increases each year. The amount is based on the length of time that someone has participated in the scheme and their salary. Some schemes base the pension on someone's pay when they retire or leave the scheme. A career-average pension is based on the average of a person's pay while they are a member of that particular scheme.

Defined Contribution Pension

A defined contribution pension builds up a pension pot and you can then draw retirement income from it. The amount in the pension depends on any charges levied, investment performance, and how much the employee and employer paid in. These pensions include workplace, personal and stakeholder pension schemes.

State pension choices

You can choose either to claim your state pension or defer it four months before you reach state pension age. If you want to defer, you don't have to do anything as the pension will be deferred automatically until you claim it. If you defer, the state pension will increase by 1 per cent for every nine weeks that it is deferred.

Most defined benefit pension schemes have a retirement age of 65. If your scheme allows, you can take the pension earlier, but this can reduce the pension quite considerably. Depending on the scheme, you might be able to defer taking the pension and then you might receive a higher income when you do take it. When you take your pension, you will have to decide whether to take some of it as tax-free cash. You can take roughly up to a quarter of the value of pension benefits in this way. Reducing the amount of tax-free cash you take might increase the amount of income you receive. You can also transfer a defined benefit pension to a defined contribution pension, which enables you to access the pension more flexibly. However, it is essential to get advice from a reputable independent financial adviser as it might mean relinquishing other valuable benefits and they can advise you accordingly.

With a defined contribution pension, when you reach 55 (or younger, if you are in poor health), you have freedom over what to do with your pension pot. However, the longer you leave your pot to continue growing, the more money you will have to live on in retirement – and to pay for care.

Make sure you take impartial, expert, financial advice when dealing with pensions. Pension Wise (www.pensionwise.gov.uk) is a useful website, which is impartial and backed by the government and The Money Advice Servicc (www.moneyadviceservice.org.uk) has a useful calculator, which helps you to work out what your pension might be worth in retirement.

CHAPTER SIX

Choosing Care

Traditionally, families lived physically close to one another and caring for frail relatives was simpler as there were plenty of family members to keep an eye on them. Today, however, many families are more dispersed nationally and internationally as people move to study, work, find affordable housing, or retire. It is not uncommon for siblings to live at opposite ends of the country, or even in different countries, and they will inevitably lead busy lives with families of their own. Older people generally expect to be cared for by their offspring, as they cared for their own relatives, and can suffer huge disappointment when this turns out to be impossible. And in turn, siblings often endure feelings of guilt.

Talking about the various care options within the family as early as possible will help. Ideally, it is good to discuss future care long before it might ever be needed – preferably around retirement – but realistically, this rarely happens. But when the issue of the need for some form of care for your older relative does arise, discuss it with them and with your siblings (if you have siblings) and agree on a course of action which can be planned and shared as equitably and sensibly as possible. This might include talking to your relative's GP and social services, making the home safer with the help of an occupational therapy expert, installing assistive technology such as personal alarms, organising a befriending service, arranging day care visits and using voluntary community transport options to avoid isolation.

However, whatever you do, you do not want to press gang your relative into agreeing to care. Understanding their concerns and assessing their needs can be a slow and frustrating process, but you must be patient and listen to their worries. So it really helps to think ahead and agree on a choice of options to present to your relative/s. If you and your siblings – and possibly the GP – are all expressing similar worries and recommending solutions in a positive way, it will go some way to providing reassurance for your relative. Having a range of care options to discuss may allay their natural fears of losing their independence and mean that they feel more involved in the decision-making process, thus becoming less anxious. Whatever happens, be patient and be prepared to revisit conversations regularly.

A family meeting may be a good time to consider organising a care assessment (see pages 70–73 for full details) and Legal Power of Attorney (see pages 36–40 for full details), so some, or all, of the family can make decisions on behalf of the relative/s. This can provide peace of mind for your loved one, because someone they trust will be making decisions for them. When it comes to care options, conflict often arises when adult siblings do not agree on the care needs of their older relative. Long-standing family arguments, resentments and old patterns of behaviour can interfere with rational thinking. If siblings cannot agree about how much care a relative needs, or about whether the relative needs care at all, then it might be advisable to seek expert guidance from outside the family. This could be done via your relative's GP or via your own GP. You can ask social services to organise a care assessment at your relative's home. It is hard to argue that no care is needed when healthcare professionals give their objective view and can provide definitive answers to your and your relative's questions and concerns. Seeking advice early on may help to avoid unhelpful and unnecessary family fights.

Another common problem is when one particular sibling becomes the main caregiver – according to Carers UK and other international studies this is often a daughter, or the sibling living closest to their relatives. The lack of help and offers to share the load by other family members can cause great resentment and anger among siblings, some of whom feel they are the only one pulling their weight, and others of whom feel guilty that they live too far away, or cannot manage to do more due to work commitments. Pecking orders and old habits die hard within families, but if siblings are not helping, then the main caregiver must insist on help. We all make the mistake of presuming that everyone sees and understands the problem as we do, but sometimes, you just have to spell it out and ask for specific help. Suggest practical ways they can help. Even if they do not live nearby, there are plenty of things they can do to help your relative, such as paying bills, arranging internet shopping and researching care options. Importantly, they could have your relative to stay for short periods so that you get some much-needed respite. Children should also be encouraged to become more involved. They can visit their grandparents, help with household chores and gardening, and even help to get them online.

Anne lived five minutes away from her mother, Beryl, who was very demanding. Beryl expected Anne to come over every day – and not just to pop in, but to stay to chat, take her shopping and help her with household chores. Anne was effectively running two houses – her own and her mother's. She was the one who took her mother to the doctor's, the dentist, the chiropodist and physiotherapist. She had two brothers, one of whom lived 10 miles away, and the other who lived in Holland. Neither visited their mother very often and when they did, they usually only came over for an hour or so, or for a couple of days once a year in the case of the Dutch-dwelling sibling. Anne grew increasingly resentful. It had always been this way. As the only daughter, her brothers just expected her to shoulder the burden of Beryl's care as she had always been expected to clear up after meals when they were children, while her brothers disappeared into their bedrooms, or out to play football. Beryl seemed to think this was acceptable too and told Anne to stop moaning about it. Her brothers were busy with their work and families – as if Anne wasn't!

In the end, Anne snapped after a particularly fraught week with her mother. She fired off an email to her brothers, accusing them of a lack of interest in their mother and total selfishness in relation to herself. Her brother in Holland emailed back to say that she was being totally unrealistic if she expected him to take all his holiday just to come home to look after his mother. Further angry emails were exchanged and this brother did not visit his mother for over a year.

Anne's other brother, however, reacted very differently. He called her on the phone and they had a long chat about how she felt and how difficult it was for her being at Beryl's constant beck and call. Her brother agreed to make more of an effort and to visit a couple of times a week and to call Beryl every day for a chat. He also agreed to sort out her insurance, TV licence and the other paperwork, which took up so much of Anne's time. Anne felt some of the burden had been lifted from her shoulders and her brother was happy to help. He hadn't realised how stressed Anne was feeling until she told him and felt guilty about not having noticed this for himself.

'Sometimes,' says Anne, 'you just have to spell out clearly exactly how you feel. Regardless of the outcome, at least you've made your feelings plain. I feel better for it, even though my older brother took it the wrong way. I think being so far away makes it hard for him to really understand and he just thinks I'm whining. I'm not angry with him – just disappointed.'

If family disputes are too complicated to manage within the family, then maybe you should consider organising some extra home care for your relative, so that you are not shouldering all the work. Whatever happens, do not feel guilty. It is important, but not necessarily easy, to avoid becoming so focused on your older relative's needs that you forget to look after yourself and pay less attention to your partner, children and friends. You only have so many hours in a day and you can only ever just do your best.

Care options

There are several options when it comes to choosing care. You can choose care at home, or in specialised care accommodation, where there are a number of different options depending on the older person's needs. One further alternative is to take your relative to live with you in your own home, or within a 'granny flat' at your property. Whichever option you choose, it is essential to consider the needs and requirements of the older person, the implications for you and your family, the costs involved and how these costs will be met.

Care assessments

Normally, a care assessment is required before any services can be provided by the social services department of a local authority, but if the need is urgent, the local authority can provide help without carrying out the assessment. The local authority uses the community care assessment to decide whether a person needs a community care service and, if they do, whether it can be provided by the local authority. The assessment should result in an effective care plan being drawn up. A wide range of services could be needed, from aids and adaptations in the older person's own home to care workers coming to their home, or residential care.

The purpose of the assessment is to find out what the person's needs and circumstances are and what support they need. It is good practice for individuals and their carers to be involved fully in their own assessments and care planning. The person seeking support should be at the centre of the decision-making process that determines what services they need from the local authority and how their needs will be met. This is referred to as personalisation. The assessment may include finding out about present living arrangements, current arrangements for care, health problems and disabilities, current concerns and how they want to be supported. This should include the older person detailing the types of services they are looking for and how they want the support to be arranged. It will also consider any specific concerns of relevant family carers, so you should attend these assessments with your relative.

It is helpful to write down any important points before the assessment so you can input your concerns and do not forget any issues you want to raise. Assessments may involve a professional person, who will visit your relative and any carer, such as yourself, to establish what needs the person has. The person in need may be asked to complete a questionnaire about their requirements, which is often called a self-assessment questionnaire and can be part of the process of a fuller assessment. People with dementia can be given assistance when filling in self-assessment forms to ensure that all of their needs are considered.

A single assessment procedure ensures that older people's needs for community care services, healthcare and any other services, such as housing, will be assessed using just one procedure, although it may be spread over several visits. This should lessen the need for repeat assessments and for the same questions to be asked by different agencies. It should also enable professionals from different backgrounds to get a fuller picture of the older person and to work together closely to ensure that the person receives the best possible care. In reality, this is not always the case as communication between services are not always as integrated as they should be, so as a carer, you may need to get involved and coordinate between the parties concerned. Continual chasing may be the only way for your relative to get the care they need.

The assessment is often carried out in the person's home, as this provides a clearer picture of how they are coping and what support they need. If the assessment is arranged elsewhere, it should be somewhere that is convenient for the person being assessed, and for their carer. If the person being assessed is in hospital, the local authority may also arrange for an assessor to visit their home to get a better idea of their situation before they are discharged. The local authority social services department is responsible for coordinating the assessment, but other professionals, such as doctors, nurses or representatives from other agencies or organisations, may also provide information or take part.

Once a local authority has established that there is a need to provide a community care service, they have a duty to provide that service. The local authority should not refuse to provide the service on the grounds of cost, although if there is more than one option, it is allowed to choose the most cost-effective one.

Before the assessment appointment, you should discuss the main issues with your relative so that you can both agree on the main problems together. It is important that you discuss this in advance, so that when you have the assessment, you and your relative do not contradict each other about the care which is needed, as this may result in the local authority providing inadequate care. Often an older person will insist that they do not need help when faced with the assessment, which can be frustrating, but try to be patient and understanding of the fact that they are concerned about their loss of independence.

It is essential to make a full list of medical issues and also to make a note of all the medication your relative is taking. It is a good idea to meet with your relative's GP prior to an assessment (you will probably have done so already, as they may have instigated it) to agree a comprehensive list.

It is also helpful to let the assessor know about your relative's routine. Consider the following questions:

- Are they housebound?
- Can they wash and dress themselves?
- Can they cook for themselves and carry food?
- Can they do their own shopping?
- Do they socialise regularly?
- Do they take any exercise?
- Do they have pets?
- Do they enjoy certain hobbies or activities?
- Are they familiar with the internet?
- How important is TV to them and how many hours do they spend watching it?

It is equally important to discuss their preferences in terms of care:

- Would they prefer to stay in their own home, or would they like to move to a care home?
- Would it be a good idea to move to sheltered housing or accommodation with no stairs?
- Do they have any help at home currently?

Your relative's local council will have details online, or at their offices, about the care services they provide and the eligibility criteria. It is a good idea to review these prior to the assessment so you understand how the care assessment will be conducted and what care you might expect following the assessment.

Care at home

Many people believe that care at home will be more expensive than care in a residential home, but this is not necessarily true. A care home can cost anywhere between £40,000 to £80,000 per annum and so providing care at home can be less expensive. In addition, there are real benefits to trying to keep your relative in their own home, or downsizing them to a smaller, more manageable property. They can sleep in their own bed, they know where everything is in the house and in the surrounding neighbourhood, and they can decide how they wish to live their life. However, the time may come when, if they are to continue with this lifestyle, they will need extra help, either because they are becoming generally more frail, or because they are recovering from an illness or fall. They may start to need help around the house, or someone to shop for them, or help them with daily hygiene and cooking.

Care at home can be for a few hours per week, or as a complete live-in care service, depending on need. Full live-in care will almost certainly have to be privately funded, but the first thing to do is to arrange a care assessment with your relative's GP in order to assess their needs and then for the local authority to provide a budget for care and for other assistive technology for the home as required. Alternatively, a hospital may suggest an assessment after a period of illness or accident. Any request for local authority help will require an assessment review of your relative(s). The assessments required and the potential help available varies for each local authority.

If you decide to hire a home carer yourself directly, there are a number of issues to consider. First, when you organise home care, you become an employer. This means you will need to create an employment contract and pay salary, tax and National Insurance, sick pay and holiday pay, as well as taking out public liability insurance. People organising care themselves also have the responsibility for checking eligibility to work in the UK and conducting a Disclosure and Barring Service check (DBS) (which has replaced the Criminal Records Bureau – CRB check) and ensures any potential carer is not disbarred from care work and has no unspent criminal convictions. Employers of carers are also responsible for ensuring the carer's training remains up to date. This may mean providing cover while your carer updates their skills. Carers need to be provided with clear work guidelines, including documentation and agreed processes. They should record medication taken, follow care plans and know how to provide dietary guidance or outlines for regular exercise, physiotherapy, or other treatments which fit into the daily life of the person for whom they are caring. Finally, the employer of a carer needs to have a plan for what happens if their chosen carer falls ill, or is unable to work for other reasons. A contingency for emergency cover should definitely be built into the budget for care.

An alternative is to employ staff through a care agency, who will manage the process for you for a fee. This is called managed care and, while it is more expensive, it means that the care company will take on the National Insurance, tax, training and documentation on your behalf, as well as providing cover for your regular carer.

If part-time home care is no longer enough, you may want to consider live-in home care. This is a lesser-known alternative to residential care homes, but one which is growing in popularity as a viable option for older people and their families. Live-in care provides personal carers, who live in their client's home, 24 hours a day. Everyone has different care requirements and live-in home care allows people to stay in familiar surroundings with the very highest standards of personally tailored, professional care. Live-in care can not only provide essential support, such as washing, dressing, preparing meals and help with medication, but also housekeeping and companionship too.

Many carers and nurses are specially trained to cope with particular conditions, such as dementia, Parkinson's, stroke, Multiple Sclerosis, or palliative care. Even tasks like general administration in today's digital world create all kinds of challenges and live-in carers are on hand to manage that too. Very importantly, they can also help older people enjoy some of the things in life they once did – for example, inviting friends over for lunch, or baking a cake, which is far more difficult to do in residential care.

For most people, full time care represents a significant financial outlay, but live-in fees can compare favourably with those of residential homes, especially where couples are looked after together. Where full-time care is required and a person's primary need is a health need, all of their care fees could be paid by the NHS through NHS Continuing Care. In all cases, it is sensible to talk to a financial advisor who specialises in later-life planning.

There are two models of live-in home care: full management and introductory live-in homecare. Choosing one service over the other is a matter of personal choice as one may be more appropriate for your relative, depending on an individual's personal circumstances and those of their family.

With full management, the company provides the care employee and trains its carers, overseeing all aspects of care. This often suits families with significant other demands on their time. The introductory care service is one where agencies do not employ carers directly. They are self-employed contractors responsible for their own tax and National Insurance contributions and are paid directly by clients or their families. This is appropriate for families keen to be closely involved and 'hands-on'.

Choosing the right carer at home is essential. When you interview a carer, either directly or via an agency, you may want to consider asking them the following questions:

- Can you provide the care that is needed and meet personal preferences?
- How will you respect privacy and dignity at all times?
- Have you cared for someone with similar needs to my relative?
- How will you match the most suitable care workers to the different care needs?
- Is your organisation a member of the United Kingdom Homecare Association (UKHCA) committed to complying with the UKHCA Code of Practice?
- Are you required to register with a statutory regulator and if so, are you currently registered?
- Is your organisation insured in order to protect residents' safety and interests?
- Do you interview all your care workers before offering them work?
- Do you obtain at least two written references from your care workers' previous employers?
- Do all your care workers undergo a criminal record disclosure from the Criminal Records Bureau (in England and Wales) or Disclosure Scotland (in Scotland) or Access NI (in Northern Ireland)?
- What sort of training do your care workers receive before they start work and during their employment?
- What proportion of your care workers and managers have obtained a recognised qualification in health and social care or management?
- If care isn't provided by a local council, do you have a standard contract that I can read before signing?

- How can I contact you or your agency during the day, outside office hours and in an emergency?
- What happens if my regular care worker is sick or on holiday?
- What charges, if any, will I be expected to pay?
- What payment methods are available (cheque, direct debit, etc.)?
- Is there a minimum charge if I only need a small amount of care?
- Are there any hidden extras in the prices you quote? (Prices normally include National Insurance contributions, travel expenses and any VAT payable.)

Completing an attendance allowance form

Attendance allowance is granted to those people over 65 who require personal care assistance. The application form can be very long and difficult, so it is a good idea to ask a friend or relative to plan it with you. Ensure that you have the accompanying notes in front of you, which are available from www.nidirect.gov.uk as they will assist you to fill in the form. If you can, print the notes off, as it is useful to be able to refer to them as you go along. The forms are also available in larger print and braille for those people who are vision impaired.

Speak to the relevant GP before completing the form and ask them to agree to speak to the Department for Work and Pensions (DWP) about the application if they are contacted. This will prevent unnecessary hold-ups later in the process. Provide as much detail as you can in the form. It is important to give as full a picture as possible. Specifically, when thinking about the assistance you or your relative might require, think about your relative's worst days rather than their best days so you do not underestimate the care you might need. This should include help with personal hygiene, such as washing and going to the toilet – including incontinence issues – and help with dressing and undressing, preparing food, carrying food, eating, and sorting and taking medicines. It is also important to note any mobility issues around the home, including difficulty using the stairs, getting in and out of chairs and in and out of the bath. Think about the type of aids and home adaptation that might help. In particular, you should try to assess the risk of falls. Also, consider whether there is any visual or aural impairment, or signs of dementia.

Make sure that a relative fills in the section at the end of the form, which asks for someone else's view on the situation, not the person asking for assistance, as this will help you to get a positive outcome. You can ask the GP if you do not have a relevant friend or relative who can do it for you. If you are helping your relative to fill out the form, make sure that they sign it personally, unless you have been granted Power of Attorney over them. The form must be posted, not emailed, and this includes the form which can be filled in online.

Safety at home

Home should be where we are safest, but as people age, so their risk of accident increases. Falling is the most common type of home accident for older people. One third of people over 65 and 50 per cent of all people over 80 fall annually, with resultant bone fractures, bruising and other complications, including reduced confidence. However, with certain precautions, most accidental falls can be prevented.

Make sure that their home has good lighting so that your relative can see where they are going easily. Buying long-life bulbs means they last longer and do not need to be changed as frequently. Ensure there are light switches at the top and bottom of the stairs, so that the light is always switched on when going up or down. Highlight outer edges of steps with non-slip white paint or Duct tape to make them more visible. Light dark corners in rooms and hallways to avoid tripping.

Tidy up trailing wires and clutter in walking areas and on the stairs, and use non-slip mats under rugs, in the kitchen, inside and next to the bath and on hallways and stair landings. It is a good idea to install non-slip rubber mats in the bath or shower and to fit grab handles to assist entry and exit from the bath or shower, as well as installing handrails by the toilet and stairs to aid balance and help with safe mobility. Grab rails are also useful by the front door to provide stability when opening locks.

Encourage the use of well-fitted, flat shoes or slippers when at home and avoid trailing clothes. Check carpets are not frayed and avoid using loose mats, which can easily slip underfoot. Store frequently used, everyday items in accessible places to minimise bending and stretching and invest in a set of non-slip steps so that your relative is not tempted to stand on a chair. You can also buy grabbers to reach high shelves, or items on the floor, if they have problems bending down. It is a good idea to remove casters from moveable furniture, which will make them more stable, so they can be leant against, or held onto to aid balance. Outside the house, make sure you spread salt, or sand on wet or icy steps in the winter to avoid falls.

Older people are more at risk from fire due to a poorer sense of smell, restricted or slow mobility and less resilience to the effects of smoke and burns. So make sure that you have fitted working smoke alarms on each floor of their home, preferably mains operated, or one with a 10-year battery, and test them regularly. If there are smokers in the home, try to remind them to safely extinguish cigarettes and never to smoke in bed. Follow the manufacturer's instructions when using electric blankets and have them checked regularly. The fire brigade run regular blanket testing days – you can find details of these at the Trading Standards department of your local council, or ask an electrician to come to your home to test the blanket. If an electric blanket is older than 10 years, it should be replaced.

Eric was 79 and lived alone in a flat in Battersea, London. He relied on his trusted electric blanket and used it every night without fail. Unfortunately, one night in February 2017, the blanket shorted and caught fire while he was asleep. Neighbours raised the alarm, but Eric was so badly burned that he died a few days later. The local fire brigade commented: 'Eric was one of over 5,000 people to suffer burns as a result of a house fire caused by an old electric blanket in the UK this year. We urge everyone to get their electric blanket checked every six months and to replace them regularly so that similar tragedies can be avoided.'

The main causes of accidental poisoning of people over 65 include carbon monoxide poisoning, mains gas poisoning and medicine overdose. Make sure that the home has a carbon monoxide alarm, which is in working order and checked regularly. Get annual checks on all fuel-burning boilers, fires and stoves and have chimneys and flues swept at least once every year. Contact burns to those over 65 can prove to be fatal. The main sources include radiators, electric fires and cookers.

Scalding causes many injuries. Try to encourage the use of radiator covers and be careful when purchasing electric fires and halogen hobs, which often retain heat long after they are switched off, so it is easy to burn yourself on them. Buy a cordless kettle, or one with a coiled flex, or even better, a small electric urn for instant hot water, which never has to be lifted to be poured when hot. Encourage your relative never to boil full kettles as they are difficult to lift and pour slowly to avoid splashes. Use a fireguard and ensure their nightwear is fire resistant. It is also a good idea to fit thermostatically controlled bath taps to stop water running too hot and so avoid scalding.

Exceeding prescribed drug doses is dangerous, so try to always read and carefully adhere to the instructions on the label and use pill boxes and counters to help you administer these. Many pill boxes come with helpful alarms to remind your relative to take their medicines on time, or there are now many smartphone apps which also work as helpful reminders. These can also be linked to family members so that you can remember to remind them to take their medication.

Many older people struggle to stay warm at home so wearing several thin layers of clothes rather than one thick layer can really help as bodily warmth gets trapped between the layers and provides better insulation. Clothes made with wool, cotton or fleece synthetic fibres are both light and warm. In very cold weather, bed socks and thermal underwear are useful. Electric blankets can help provide warmth, but must be well maintained and should be regularly checked and replaced if more than 10 years old. Fit draught proofing to help seal gaps around windows and doors and check that there is sufficient loft insulation to reduce heat loss. Hot water cylinders and pipes, including pipes in the loft, should be lagged. Try to keep a temperature of 21°C (70°F) in all the rooms used during the day. Many older people scrimp on the heating due to cost, but this can be fatal. There are benefits available for older people to help with heating costs as detailed on page 54. Keep the bedroom windows closed at night and in very cold weather. It is better to set the central heating to come on earlier rather than turning the thermostat up higher. It seems obvious but it's worth reminding your relative that when going out in cold weather, it is a good idea to wear a hat and in icy weather, ice grippers placed over shoes or sturdy boots can be a lifesaver in terms of preventing slips and falls – for all of us, not just older people!

Personal alarms can be very useful to provide peace of mind for older people and for their families if they are not with them at home. Many social services departments view alarms as daily living equipment and will provide them free of charge following a care assessment by an occupational therapist, or for a small weekly fee. If you are going to buy an alarm yourself, you need to consider which of the many options you want to choose. Some alarms will alert a carer, or neighbour. These include portable alarms, which are battery-powered or use pressurised gas, and can be bought from high street shops, through mail order or online. They are worn usually as a neck pendant or watch and make a high-pitched sound when triggered, which can be heard from a limited distance. Or you can choose a fixed position alarm, which has a fixed transmitter and receiver and is operated by a pull cord or similar trigger, sending a high-pitched sound to alert anyone within a limited distance. Some systems can be designed to release door locks automatically if activated, to allow a friend or neighbour to enter the home when the alarm is triggered.

You can also get alarms linked to a central call centre, which will alert you by phone if your relative is in distress. Portable transmitters and portable receivers allow both you and the person you are looking after to wear the device around your neck or wrist. This makes it easier for you to be aware of when the alarm is triggered. It is suitable for a limited range, such as when either of you is in the house or garden.

Top tip: Be aware that many older people hate wearing these devices, particularly those with obvious neck pendants. Devices worn around the wrist can be far less obtrusive, but even then, your relative may not wear it and then the alarm is useless. Do make sure that you choose an alarm which is not dependent on the user wearing the device if your relative is not keen as it will not provide the safety element you seek and will be a waste of money.

You may want an alarm that can monitor the person you are looking after if you are in another room of the house. There are several options, including one-way intercom, which is a portable system, similar to a baby monitor, which allows sounds or speech to be transmitted one-way only. You can also get fall alarms, which are portable and activated when the person wearing it falls to an angle of 20 degrees or more and lies without moving for eight seconds. A signal is then sent to a portable pager, or an autodial alarm telephone is activated. Movement monitors are mainly used at night and can alert you to epileptic seizures by detecting movement or monitoring vital signs. An alarm is triggered by sensors.

Wandering alarms alert you when a person strays. This alarm is activated by pressure sensors located in a bedside mat or doorway, or when someone gets out of bed. Some alarms are worn and trigger a warning alarm if the person goes through a door fitted with an antenna. A hypothermia alarm is used to monitor the ambient temperature. The alarm is triggered if the temperature falls below a designated level. You can also get auto-dialler systems, which send voice or text messages without needing a phone if someone falls.

You might also enhance security via a keyless door entry system, which helps people who have difficulty using keys to open their front door. They are especially suitable for those who have to let in carers, or would benefit from instant home access in case of emergency. They work via a remote control, which fits comfortably in the palm of the hand for those with arthritis.

Downsizing

It is widely acknowledged that moving house is among the most stressful experiences in life. However, this may need to be considered as people age for a variety of reasons, such as health conditions, changes in mobility, bereavement, or simply to be nearer to family, or to have a smaller, more manageable home. There may also be financial considerations, such as needing to fund care.

Downsizing may come as a very welcome and positive change for some, but it will necessitate de-cluttering and disposing of collections, furniture and personal items, which will inevitably be stressful for many. This is emotionally and physically draining work for carers as well, so take care of yourself and be sure to get the support you need to stay positive and well yourself, as you manage estate agents, solicitors and your relative about what stays and what goes. It is often emotional for family carers too, if the home being sold is that of their childhood.

Some people choose to downsize to a retirement home or village, which is an increasingly popular option. Most of these require you to buy a property and many of them provide a warden on call in case of emergency. Some provide a broad range of assisted living and care options, depending on the care required.

Care homes

Types of care home are many and varied and it is, as ever, important to consider the needs of the older person before deciding on the right home. However, critically, it is important to think not only about their current needs, but also future needs, hence minimising the need to keep moving. Homes range from those offering care accommodation with meals and cleaning to those offering nursing or specialist care options for dementia. Many homes offer a range of care so that if health deteriorates, the home can still look after someone's needs without the requirement to move again.

Choosing a care home

When choosing a care home, there are a number of important issues to consider. Before you start shortlisting any potential care homes, it is a good idea to sit down with your relative (assuming they are still well enough to have such discussions) and agree what is important to them, and to you and your siblings. You should consider issues such as location – is it an area your relative is familiar with if they intend to go shopping or visit friends and is it convenient for family and friends to visit? You should also consider what facilities the home offers and critically, if they offer specialist care for specific health problems – current and possibly future. It is a good idea to involve siblings as well.

You can search for homes on the Care Quality Commission website www.cqc.org.uk, which inspects and ranks all care homes. It is also always a good idea to ask friends for recommendations and to check out any comments online.

Top tip: Spend time looking through the individual websites of care homes which might be of interest in order to get an idea of how they operate, what the accommodation and facilities are like and to help you to draw up a list of questions for when you visit.

Once you have made a shortlist and before you visit, call and ask to speak to the manager on the phone. Ask about what rooms they have available, about the facilities and care options and importantly, ask about fees. If they are reluctant to discuss these over the phone, persist. There is no point in going to visit if the fees are unaffordable. The home will want to know if your relative is self-funding, local authority funded, or a mixture of the two. You might not know the answer to this yet, if the assessment has not been completed. If this is the case, just explain this to the manager. Ask them to send you a brochure and written details of costs prior to visiting the home.

When you visit the home in person and while there, ask yourself a number of important questions:

- Is the home clean and tidy inside and out?
- Are there cigarette butts outside the front door and does the home smell fresh? There is no excuse for poor smell, so beware of excessive use of air freshener, which is just used to mask poor hygiene and cleaning
- Do the staff appear to be running the home to suit themselves, or for the benefit of the residents? Ask plenty of questions and you will soon find out if they really care about the residents
- Do the staff smile and stop to chat to the other residents as they show you around? They should have strong, positive relationships with the people they are looking after
- What activities are offered and how are residents encouraged to get involved? Exercise, both mental and physical, should be actively encouraged, as well as excursions beyond the confines of the home
- How open is the home management to collaboration with families? Ask how they handle complaints. If they are reluctant to answer any such questions, then be wary of the home.

Suggested questions to ask when visiting a care home:

- When is the room available/is there a waiting list? You must ask to see all available rooms and the bathrooms

- Can your relative bring their own furniture? How much stuff can they bring with them?
- What levels of care are available?
- Does the home use all permanent workers or are some agency staff? If so, what is the ratio of permanent to agency carer workers? Ideally, you want a home where the majority of care workers are permanent to ensure consistent levels of care
- What is the care provision at night?
- If your relative's condition should deteriorate, can the home provide adequate care, or would your relative have to move?
- What is food like? Ask to visit the dining room during meal times and look at the menus
- Can your relative eat in their room when they prefer to?
- What social activities are on offer?
- Are there set visiting times for guests and are children welcome?
- Can guests eat at the home and stay overnight? What does this cost?
- What security is there to stop residents from wandering, or trespassers coming in?
- Are pets allowed and does the home have a resident pet(s)?
- How can your relative store their valuables?
- What is the complaints procedure?
- How much are the fees and what do they include and exclude?
- Are fees due weekly or monthly and in advance or in arrears?
- If relevant, how are NHS-funded nursing care payments accounted for in the fee structure? (They should be deducted from the overall fee)
- How often are fees reviewed and how much did they increase by year on year over the last five years? How much notice does the home give for fee increases?
- Are residents tied into the care home contract for a minimum period?
- Is there a deposit and is it refundable? What are the terms?
- Is there a limit to how long a resident can be absent from the care home before their contract is affected?

- How much notice must your relative give if they want to leave and would they be entitled to a pro-rata refund of any fees already paid? How much notice does the home give if they wish your relative to leave?

Once you have gone through the process of selecting suitable care accommodation and you and your relative have decided to make the move, you will need to start making arrangements to transport their possessions and prepare for the movers. You may need to put their current property on the market. If so, it is a good idea to contact at least three local estate agents to get an idea of the market value and fees involved and consider the way they will market the property and what the houses are currently selling for within the area within that price range. You should also source a solicitor to act for you on the sale and purchase, if they are buying a retirement or care property.

Top tip: It is better to use a solicitor not recommended by the estate agent to avoid a conflict of interest.

If renting, the notice period that you will have to give your current landlord needs consideration. Work this in with the date your relative will be able to move. You can check this on the tenancy agreement, or by contacting your landlord/lettings agent.

Once you know the date that your relative will be moving, it is important to let providers know and to give them your relative's new address. People you will need to contact may include electricity, gas, the bank/building society, pension providers, water companies, and telephone and broadband providers. Utilities will require relevant meter readings. Do not forget also to notify their GP, dentist and optician, as well as the council and DVLA. You may want to consider arranging for mail to be redirected for a time. This can be useful if you have not had the time to tell all your relative's contacts about their change of address, or you have forgotten to contact someone. Try and arrange this well beforehand, which you can do easily through the Post Office (note there is a fee for this redirect service).

Think about what items might move to the care home with your relative and what is already there. If using a removals company, make sure they are reputable by checking that they are a member of the British Association of Removers (https://bar.co.uk). It is best to get at least two quotations for the move and decide how much help you will need.

It is a good idea to arrange a home visit with your relative to their new home at least a week before they move in to check where things are and to familiarise yourself and your relative with the layout and facilities. Take the time to chat to staff and residents and ask any further questions you may have prior to moving in. They often have some helpful tips about what to and what not to bring with you.

The role of social services

Social services will help with specific equipment to assist someone to move around the home and with assistive technology items to help with other issues around the home. They will also assist with at home care and provide care home services if required. They run day care centres, community activities and provide transport. They can also offer legal and financial support.

In terms of assistive technology, this might mean adapting the bathroom to install a shower rather than a bath, attaching grip rails by the toilet, ensuring the stair lighting is adequate, or even providing raised toilet seats, or tools to help with opening jars and tins. For mobility problems, hoists can be supplied, as well as walking frames and wheelchairs. There might also be a requirement for in-house monitors to prevent wandering or falls. A social worker and occupational therapist will help you to get the required items, usually as part of a care assessment (more details on pages 70–73).

Social services can also provide carers to come into your relative's home and help with washing, dressing, cleaning and laundry, eating and getting in and out of bed. You may be provided with a personal budget to choose your own care. If your relative can no longer manage at home, social services will work with you on how to move them to a suitable care home, dependent on their needs.

Social services can provide transport to help older people to get out and about to meet like-minded others in community centres. Such centres are invaluable to many older people to prevent loneliness and isolation. Additionally, the local authority may run volunteering schemes to help your relative to remain active and engaged within the community. Your relative's local authority should have a full list of activities, which will be available online. Day centres provide food, company and activities, which many older people will struggle to access if they always remain at home. They can also provide daily respite care for family carers. Your relative's local authority should have a full list of day care centres.

The funding of all of the above should be discussed with your relative as part of the care assessment provided by the local authority. If your relative has an ongoing health condition, they might be eligible for NHS Continuing Care (see also pages 59–62).

Caring from a distance

Caring from a distance occurs when families live apart from a relative who might need assistance. This situation is of increasing concern to a significant percentage of the UK population. Caring from a distance can mean living relatively close by, or far away. The travelling time, even for short distances, can add stress to a carer's life and often increases their guilt if they do not visit regularly. In addition, these days, people are far less likely to know and, therefore, to rely on, their neighbours for help. Modern technology leads to longer working hours, which older people often find hard to understand. Older people expect to be cared for as they cared for their own relatives, but this is often not possible, so expectations on both sides are sometimes not met. Distance carers can feel that they never seemingly do enough according to other family members and themselves, particularly when coping with crises.

It does help to have conversations early on, but this is not always easy and is often avoided. However, having conversations with relatives and siblings early on can be of enormous benefit. Talk to them about their views on possible future care, financial planning, possible downsizing, granting Power of Attorney, making a will and even funeral wishes. When a crisis hits, you will be better prepared and more able to help productively and quickly. When someone does get older and needs help, there are plenty of ways you can help from a distance. Communication is at the core. Send photographs by email or post to keep them in touch with how everyone in your family is getting on and what they are up to. Set your relative up with a laptop or iPad if they can be persuaded to try one. Then you can email each other and talk via Skype. Setting up Skype is easy to do and you can talk face-to-face with your relative, even if you cannot be physically there. Skype is easy for older people to grasp as they just have to hit a button, see a name, press that and they can talk to you. See page 259 for help with terminology.

In addition, you and your relative can use the internet to help, for shopping and for entertainment. You can help your relative with the shopping from wherever you are by setting up a weekly online food delivery for them. Talk to them about what they would like to order each week and let them order online, or do it for them, depending on their situation. You can always include a bunch of flowers or chocolates as a surprise treat. Some online supermarkets have a minimum £40 spend, so if that is too high for a relative living alone, you could try Milk & More (www.milkandmore.co.uk), which has no minimum spend and delivers a range of basic food items to your door via the milkman.

You can also consider opening a taxi account for your relative if they need to get out and cannot drive or manage public transport. Set the number up on speed dial on their phone so they can book a taxi easily and not worry about paying. Taxi accounts sound expensive, but can be very useful for occasional trips out and can help prevent people becoming housebound. If your relative drives irregularly, a taxi account can be cheaper than keeping a car and paying for insurance, tax, maintenance and repairs. You can often negotiate a rate with a local taxi service for regular usage. The Royal Voluntary Service (www.royalvoluntaryservice.org.uk) can provide door-to-door community transport services so that older people can maintain a good quality of life and stay connected to their local communities.

Similarly, travel assistance is available on trains and planes. Registering as disabled (see pages 143–147) can give an older person access to parking and a range of discounts. Note that not all disabled badges work in all places, so be careful or you may be fined. Help your relative to travel to you by arranging train travel, so they do not have to drive. You can book tickets online, which can be sent directly to them. All airlines offer special assistance for the older person if organised in advance, including accompanying them through the airport and transporting them to and from the aircraft.

If you are worried about falls or accidents within the home, you can get them a care alarm so that you can be contacted quickly in an emergency. Get them to carry a mobile phone with them and add essential numbers, just in case. See page 26 for emergency card details. Simplified phones with extra-large numbers, such as those made by Doro, can make using a mobile very easy for older people, who might not be able to work a smartphone.

Make sure their GP has your emergency numbers on their records. If possible, set up a visit rota with friends and family to make sure there is some regular contact happening throughout the week. Thousands of older people in the UK go months on end without speaking to another person and loneliness kills. Regular communication is so important.

If you feel your relative is getting a bit isolated, why not suggest some new activities (depending on their health and mobility needs), such as volunteering, or learning new skills at the University of the Third Age (www.u3a.org.uk), which is a national organisation providing classes specifically designed to help people to study in their later years.

Hospital discharge

If your relative has been in hospital, it should be good news when they are ready to come home, but sometimes, managing their discharge from hospital can be a real worry, particularly if you live far away. Hospitals must have a plan to help your relative to go home safely from there. If you are unsure what these plans are, you must ask, as every hospital will follow different procedures. They should have a team co-ordinating the discharge and they may also involve a social worker. A discharge should only be arranged when the patient is well enough to go home and the doctors are satisfied that this is the case, but also it is imperative that the patient has sufficient care at home so that they can manage and continue their recovery. If you or your relative do not feel they should be discharged, you must discuss this with the doctors and other medical staff. Similarly, if you do not believe that your relative can manage at home, you must ensure you are happy with the arrangements the hospital are suggesting.

Often older people will try to discharge themselves because they want to go home. The doctors should prevent this, but sometimes they can persuade them that they are better than they are and that they can manage at home, just because they are desperate to leave hospital. You must work with the hospital staff to ensure they have the full picture. You and your relative should be involved and informed about all arrangements. To be discharged, your relative should be judged to be medically well enough and have been assessed for care needed at home. They should have been given a written care plan detailing the support they will receive and assured that this support is ready for them when they leave. Your relative should never be discharged in the middle of the night, or without adequate arrangements for transport, but sadly, this does happen. The Royal Voluntary Service also runs a home from hospital scheme, which can help ensure that an older person can return home safely after a hospital stay. Some areas also give practical and social support to older people when they need it most during a hospital stay, by providing friendship, companionship and support through conversation.

Discharge/care plans are usually arranged by a key worker, or discharge coordinator, who is a nurse or other healthcare professional. This person should be your relative's main point of contact during their stay in hospital. Following discharge, they might require ongoing care from various organisations and healthcare professionals. If they do, their key worker should manage the arrangements for when they go home. In order to prepare an effective discharge plan, the key worker should check their mobility levels, including managing stairs, their ability to wash, dress and make food and assess whether help is required with these issues. Depending on the needs of the patient, their key worker will liaise with social workers, physiotherapists, occupational therapists, speech therapists, mental health nurses and dieticians. The key worker should take time to ensure all adequate resources are in place before discharge takes place. A social worker may be called in to arrange at home care. If intermediate care is required, this can be arranged free of charge for six weeks without the need for full assessment and regardless of savings and income. If needs have changed significantly, they may need to be assessed for ongoing care support.

A discharge plan should include support and treatment needed on an ongoing basis, details of who is responsible for providing care and their contact details, plus details of who is coordinating the overall plan, when and how often the care will be provided and how the care will be monitored and reviewed. It should also provide a list of emergency contacts and any relevant information about who is paying for which services. A care plan could include community care services, following an assessment, NHS Continuing Care, for those with very severe and complex healthcare needs, NHS-funded nursing care, for those who need to be cared for in a nursing home, intermediate care, which is short-term care free of charge for a maximum of six weeks at home, or palliative care. It may also detail requirements for special mobility equipment, such as wheelchairs, beds or adaptations for daily living and possible support from voluntary agencies.

When discharged, you and your relative should have a copy of their care plan. Transport should be arranged and their carer, if they have one, should know they are coming home. Their GP should know they are being discharged and they should be given the medicine and any other supplies they need. They should also know how to use any assisted technology or mobility aids as necessary, should have suitable clothes and shoes to wear and have keys and money.

Mabel, aged 85, was sent home by taxi at 11 o'clock in the evening. She was in a confused state and had a catheter still in place. There was no one at home to receive her as the hospital had not notified her family that they were sending her home. Mabel had no food at home and the heating was off. When a neighbour noticed that her front door was open the next day, they found her lying in her overcoat on the bed with her catheter pulled out and blood all over the sheets. An ambulance was called and Mabel ended up back in hospital for a further two weeks due to a severe urinary tract infection.

Care complaints

Most people have a positive experience of the care they receive, but problems sometimes occur and you may wish to make a complaint. Whether the care is provided at home, or in a care home, or if you have bought a care product, such as a mobility aid, it is important to know your rights.

Care homes and home care providers are regulated in England by the Care Quality Commission (CQC), in Scotland by the Care Inspectorate, in Wales by the Care and Social Service Inspectorate and in Northern Ireland by the Regulation and Quality Improvement Authority. They are all responsible for ensuring that the care someone receives, whether it is provided at home or in a care home, meets national minimum standards. These standards are not just guidelines. Providers have a legal obligation to make sure people are safe, comfortable and treated with respect. And if things go wrong, you have a legal right to complain.

In England, Wales and Northern Ireland, regulatory bodies are responsible for checking that every registered care provider meets important standards of quality and safety, but their duties do not include dealing with individual complaints about providers' services. However, the Care Inspectorate in Scotland will investigate complaints against providers and has the power to enforce recommendations or even revoke a provider's operating licence.

You can clear up many problems by having an informal chat with a member of staff or the manager of the care home or service, but if that does not get a result, or if the member of staff or manager is the problem, you will need to make a formal complaint. By law, all registered health and social care service providers must have a complaints procedure that you can ask to see. It should have been explained to you when your relative moved in, or took up a particular service. Ask for a copy of the provider's complaints policy so you know what to do.

If you are still not satisfied with the response from your care provider, and your local council pays for all or some of your care, you should complain through their social services department. They will investigate the complaint and take any appropriate actions. If you fund and arrange your own care, you should take your complaint directly to the Local Government Ombudsman and/or the Health Service Ombudsman, but only after your care provider has been given a reasonable opportunity to put matters right. In England, the Local Government Ombudsman should be your first port of call if you feel you need to elevate a complaint made to your local council about residential or nursing care. The Health Service Ombudsman can only consider complaints about the NHS. In England, contact the Local Government Ombudsman. In Scotland, contact the Scottish Public Service Ombudsman. In Wales, contact the Public Services Ombudsman for Wales and for Northern Ireland, contact the Northern Ireland Ombudsman. If you think your case involves criminal negligence or fraud, you should speak to a solicitor and if you believe there are serious criminal acts taking place, such as physical abuse, theft or other forms of criminal activity, you should contact the police.

Do not withhold payment for a care product or service without first getting professional advice about your rights and responsibilities. Contact your local authority if the care home is run by them, or get advice from your local Citizens Advice Bureau (www. citizensadvice. org.uk). You can also get advice from charities, or support organisations, such as Age UK (www.ageuk.org.uk) and Action on Elder Abuse (www. elderabuse.org.uk). Keep copies of any emails and letters you send, and make sure you use recorded delivery for anything you post.

When you buy a care product, the law gives you certain rights that protect you if it is faulty or not fit for purpose and this includes equipment or aids to help with mobility or daily tasks. If your council has arranged for and purchased a care product for you, report it to them and they should replace it. If you bought a care product directly, go back to the retailer to ask for a refund or replacement. If you do not get a satisfactory result, contact your local Citizens Advice Bureau for help in taking matters further. If you bought a product or service with a credit card and the retailer is being difficult, you may get help from your credit card provider. Contact them directly to see what they can do.

If you have purchased a financial care product and you are not satisfied with the service, ask for a copy of the company's complaints procedure and launch an official complaint directly with them. Firms regulated by the Financial Conduct Authority are legally obliged to have one. If you do not get a satisfactory outcome, contact the Financial Ombudsman Service to complain. If the Financial Ombudsman Service has considered your complaint and you are still unhappy, you can take the matter to court. However, bear in mind that, in most cases, the court is likely to agree with the Financial Ombudsman Service's decision, and it could be a lengthy and costly process.

CHAPTER SEVEN

The Effective Use of Technology

Today's society is more connected than ever before. The vast majority of the population now uses the internet, smartphones and social media to communicate and keep in touch with friends. In the UK alone, 38 million people use Facebook. Yet, at the same time, there are around one million older people who have not spoken to a friend, neighbour or family member for at least a month. Loneliness is the biggest killer in older people due to the real mental and physiological problems it creates – it is a very real problem.

There is a sharp divide in the uptake of the use of technology across generations. Those people who could benefit most from technology are least likely to have access to it, or have the confidence to try it. In addition, as technology becomes more pervasive in general society, we are seeing a breakdown of traditional forms of social interaction. For example, younger people are now less inclined to make phone calls, preferring instead short instant messaging, which further isolates the older population.

The good news is that it is never too late to learn how to use a computer or tablet and a large proportion of the UK now has superfast broadband, which makes booking holidays, shopping for groceries, streaming online films, or speaking to the family on Skype or FaceTime so easy and a great way to combat loneliness. More and more older people are getting interested in using computers, because they want to stay in touch with their families and we must do our best to encourage their engagement with technology – even in the most reluctant.

Computers

Fortunately for many older people, there are family members and friends who will help them learn to use a computer, particularly grandchildren, who tend to understand technology better than the rest of us. If your relative does not have that kind of help to hand, there are classes available which can familiarise them with the internet and email. Even if they do not type very fast, or are a little bit unsure of what they are doing, older people can see the benefit of connecting with their loved ones and with people they know all over the world simply by clicking a button. Increasingly, older people have been joining social networking sites too, so that they can make new friends and reconnect with old ones.

Computers can also transform how older people shop and how they entertain themselves. If someone is less mobile, computers can provide them with access to a whole new world, where they can find shopping, information, entertainment and contacts online. Computers can also be used to promote life-long learning, as older people can research areas of interest, or take online courses.

How to encourage an older person to try a computer

By far the biggest problem with regard to using technology for older people is lack of confidence. Many older people encountering computers for the first time believe that it will all be far too difficult for them to make sense of at their age and therefore it is easier not to try. The best advice to combat this reluctance is not to call a machine a computer or a laptop, but just to show them what it does.

Matt went to see his grandma and took his tablet with him.

'Hi, Grandma, let me show you something amazing.'

'What is it?'

'Oh, it's this really easy thing. Just look.' He opens his tablet. 'You see this square here?' He points to the Skype icon.

'Yes,' says his grandma.

'Just press it.'

His grandma reaches over and taps the blue icon. Skype's home page appears with Matt's contacts.

'Now press Mum's name,' says Matt.

His grandma does so and she hears a ringing noise, followed by her daughter's face appearing on the screen.

'Hi, Mum,' laughs her daughter.

'Hello, what are you doing in there?'

'Oh, well, I'm talking to you. If you like, Matt can get you a screen too and then you can call and talk face-to-face whenever you like.'

'Well, I never! How clever! Matt, when can you get one for me? Can I call your aunt as well?'

'Yes, of course. You can call her in Australia. You just have to get the time difference right!'

One feature of computer applications which older people often find difficult is mastering the large number of details that must be remembered in order to accomplish tasks, such as logging on, opening up specific programmes and managing passwords. Each detail is small in itself, but all must be learned in order to make use of the software correctly. Once the steps have been clarified, however, they can then use strategies to remember what to do, such as having reminder sheets by the keyboard, or making good use of online help facilities, which can be saved on the main screen as an icon. There are also a number of simplified software applications, which minimise the steps necessary to use a computer. You can search for these online as new versions and concepts are emerging all the time.

One physical skill that many older people find very difficult at first is using the computer mouse. Many report that this problem alone has meant they have abandoned attempts to attend classes in introductory computing since they are embarrassed at their slowness in acquiring this minor, but important skill. If the mouse becomes a real problem, there are touch screen computers available, which can take away the fear of using the computer, or many older people find tablets a much easier option. However, a few hours of practice with the mouse usually solves any problems, but this must be mastered before any real applications involving using the mouse are attempted, or confidence will suffer and they may decide to give up entirely.

Learning to use the computer with other older people can help as it avoids the embarrassment the learner might feel with a younger person who knows all about the technology and struggles to understand why other people just don't get it. Also, having an older person as a teacher provides a constant role model and proof that the technology can, in fact, be mastered by someone who is no longer young. Check your local education authority, or other local educational groups, many of whom will run very useful beginners courses on computing. There are also a number of helpful computing books available, such as *Computing for Dummies for Seniors*. If you can persuade your older relative to embrace the computer, they will be able to live more fulfilling lives due to the access it will give them.

Tablets

The amazing thing about the iPad and other similar tablets is that they are a natural extension of the normal interface between the hand and the brain, which means that they are very straightforward for everyone to use, including older people with no previous experience of technology. It is very easy to get started using a tablet. As with computers, the best way of introducing a tablet to an older person is simply to say, 'Have you seen this?' Do not mention 4G, Wi-Fi, etc., as it can get scary and confusing, unless the person you are giving it to already understands these terms, or wants to know. Hand the tablet to them switched on with an app open on the screen and let them start looking around. Apps are designed to be very intuitive, so they will soon be able to start interacting.

It is a good idea to establish what interests your relative (e.g. arts and crafts, cooking, news, games, crosswords, etc.) and start searching from there. There are many thousands of apps available and the choice is enormous, with costs ranging from free to around £5 for more complex software. To help you to help your relative to choose, type in the keywords for what you are looking for (e.g. drawing) into the search box and let the machine find the apps for you. If you just want free apps, you can filter the search for free apps accordingly.

There are certain apps which are definitely worth putting on an older person's tablet, such as Skype and/or FaceTime, so that they can call you and chat to you live. These apps provide free unlimited face-to-face contact with anyone, or any computer anywhere in the world through Wi-Fi, as long as they are also registered with these apps. All you need is an email address and Wi-Fi or broadband. You can arrange specific times to call, so your relative is ready and expecting you.

The iPad and other tablets have a camera on the front and on the back, so it does not matter how your relative holds it when speaking to you, as they can switch easily between the two. Being able to see your relative when talking has many advantages. You can see if they look healthy and well groomed, and you can keep a regular check on them. You can also involve them more in your life by using the outward camera to show them how your garden is looking, the mess in the kids' room, etc., so they feel more involved.

YouTube is also another good app to enable your relative to view short video clips on almost anything you can imagine. It has such a diversity of content, so it really allows the user to follow what they are interested in and can be very entertaining as well, helping to pass the time. Older people can look at events from their past, on channels such as Pathé News, or view old films. Or they can learn something new, such as how to make greetings cards, or to find a new, easy recipe.

They can even choose music to listen to and sing along. YouTube also has videos on how to fix almost anything, which can take some of the stress away from the family, so if your relative is still mentally well enough to watch such videos and follow instructions, they can be very helpful.

In addition, there are many very useful medical and monitoring apps, which can help to keep older people safe in the home, helping you to keep tabs on their medication and reminding them to take it at the right time with the correct dosage.

They can also bank online, which is becoming more necessary with the closure of so many retail banking sites. Online shopping, particularly for heavy household items, can be a great help and the delivery people are usually more than happy to take the goods into the home and to help unpack, if needed.

Mobile phones

Mobile phones can be a very useful line of communication for older people and their children, both as a way of staying in touch day-to-day and as a reassuring emergency tool for the most vulnerable. Encouraging older people to agree to use a mobile phone, however, can be a difficult hurdle to overcome, especially if they have never owned one and they may think them too complex to work, or too expensive to run. They might also find it difficult to use the small buttons on a standard mobile, due to a disability, sight problems, or because of arthritic fingers, but there are many easy-to-use mobiles on the market, which are also far cheaper than smartphones. Look for phones with larger buttons (Doro produce a good range), phones which speak numbers when dialled, extra-loud speakers that have hearing aid compatibility and phones with a good battery life, so they do not need constant charging. Some also have a built-in panic button. Some are touchscreen and some are not, so you can decide which type suits your relative best.

Setting up email

Email is a great way for older people to keep in touch with family and friends. Email obviously allows you to send messages and photographs to them instantly, without needing a stamp or pen and paper, making it so much easier to communicate and keep in touch.

Many older people believe setting up an email account is complicated, but it is really very simple. There are many websites offering free email accounts, such as Google, Yahoo, AOL and Hotmail. When you visit one of these websites, you will see an option to register a new account. You need to fill in a few personal details to keep the account more secure. Any information recorded by the email providers will be kept confidential and cannot be disclosed to third parties without your or your relative's permission, so email details remain private. The address you or your relative chooses will have two parts to it: the user name and the domain name of the provider, which are separated by the @ symbol. You can choose any user name you like, as long as no one else has chosen it already. If they have, you need to add numbers or letters to make it unique to you. The domain name – such as Google or Yahoo – always stays the same depending on the chosen provider.

Choose a password your relative can remember, but which is not too easy. Your relative can make a note of it in a safe place and so can you, in case they forget it. Computers and tablets will also allow you to ask the computer to remember it for your relative. Passwords should be a combination of upper and lower case letters and numbers. It is a good idea to change your password regularly and to keep it private.

Remind your relative that when they log in to check their email, or to write a message, they will be asked to type in their email address and password, unless these details have been saved so they come up automatically. They should never save these details on a shared computer as other people can then access their email account. It is a good idea to save passwords when you help your relative to set these up initially, so they do not have to remember the details each time. Sites such as Last Pass will issue a different password for each site and remember it for you, which keeps everything secure and much simpler. All you then need to do is remember one master password. It is important to remind your relative not to give out their email address to anyone who they do not want to contact them as they may end up receiving unwanted junk mail. It is also a good idea to help them to unsubscribe from any unwanted sites every so often.

Once your relative has logged into their email account with their email address and password, they will be able to read their messages and choose to send messages to others. To do this, you can copy out this set of instructions for them to follow:

1) Type the email address of the person you want to send an email to into the box at the top marked 'To'.
2) The 'From' box will fill itself in with your email address.
3) Create a title for your message in the box marked subject. In the large box underneath, type in your message.
4) When you have finished writing your message, click on the button marked 'Send' and your message will be sent over the internet.

You might find that ads and other unwanted emails start appearing in your Inbox. If ever you are unsure about a message, delete it rather than click on it. If it is a scam email and you click on it, it can give the sender access to your email addresses and they can in turn send spam to all your contacts, send you more spam and possibly create a virus in your computer. It is always better just to block them, or delete them if you are unsure.

You can also check whether an email looks genuine by clicking on the email address it has been sent from as this usually gives a good indication of whether or not the email is real. Fake email addresses are normally self-evident, with spelling mistakes, or using the name of a random person, rather than the company it pretends to be from. If in doubt, do not open it and just delete it.

Avoiding scams

Unfortunately, there are many unscrupulous individuals who prey on all of us, but older people can be a particular target. Scams can happen online, on the phone, or at the door. The general rule to follow is that if something sounds too good to be true, it probably is too good to be true, so be suspicious. If your relative is offered a deal, whether by phone, or face-to-face, or even online, they should never make decisions immediately. Encourage them to talk to you first about any offers or deals and to take time to consider the offer. If they are keen to progress, it often makes sense to consult an independent party and take legal and/or financial advice before moving forward. Remind your relative not to get distracted by 'any time limited' offers, or special 'sign up now' deals. Scammers like to pressurise older people.

You or your relative must check the credentials of any company or individual before handing over any money, or signing anything. This is best carried out online, as then you will be able to check out multiple sources and even find out via blogs if anyone has been scammed by these organisations before. Beware of glowing testimonials as they may be false. If your relative does not have internet access, or is not familiar with these types of searches, get them to ask somebody else to do it for them.

Banking and personal details are very valuable, so your relative needs to do all they can to protect them. Remind them that they should never give any personal details to someone they do not know, or do not trust, whatever they say and however they approach them, i.e. by phone, on the doorstep or online. Impress upon them that the bank will never call and ask for bank details, so if someone does ask for them, it will be bogus. Some scammers demand payment for products or services in gift vouchers rather than cash and this should always ring alarm bells. No reputable company asks for payment by this method. Sometimes, your relative may receive requests online by email to send money to someone who is in distress, or financial difficulty abroad. Whatever the circumstances, never send money abroad, even if it is an email from someone you know, as this is almost always still a scam. When using the internet, remind your relative always to go directly to the website they want and not through a link from another site, as this might provide access to their details.

The following case study is typical of the type of fraud perpetrated on older people and was recently highlighted by the Financial Ombudsman:

Mr H took a call from someone who said they were the police. He was told that his debit cards had been compromised. Mr H was told to call his bank to check what the 'police officer' had said was true. Mr H didn't realise at the time that the fraudster was still on the line and that when he thought he was calling the bank, the call was actually diverted to the fraudster, who got Mr H to disclose personal security information. He was asked to key his PIN into the phone for verification. And while he was still on the phone to the person he thought worked for his bank, a 'courier' arrived to take his bank cards away for security reasons. Mr H soon started to feel that something was not right and contacted his bank again the following day – his real bank, this time. They confirmed that a significant sum had been removed from his savings account and more money had been withdrawn at cash machines. The bank said they could not refund the money because Mr H had been negligent in giving away confidential information.

Protecting your relative's home address is very important. If they begin to receive mail for someone they do not recognise at their address, you or they should open it and find out why it has been sent. Always shred or tear up any documents which have your relative's address and personal details on them before they go into the bin or recycling, especially banking and finance information, as unscrupulous people rifle through recycling bins looking for such personal details to use. Remind your relative never to reply to unsolicited texts, e.g. those asking about accidents or PPI, even to reply STOP, as that can also be a scam. Just delete them.

Register all your relative's phones and mail addresses to stop unsolicited calls and mail via the Telephone Preference Service (www.tpsonline.org.uk/tps) and the Mail Protection Service (www.mpsonline.org). This will go a long way to stopping junk and scam mail. You can also block callers on a relative's mobile phone and landline, if they have the right type of handset which allows numbers to be blocked. It is also vital to keep their computer's anti-virus and security programmes up-to-date.

Above all, if you or your relative has been a victim of a scam, or suspect a scam, you must report it immediately to the police. You should also contact Action Fraud 0300 123 2040, or visit their website https://www.actionfraud.police.uk.

Technology to assist care

Technology can assist with care within the home in many ways. Whether it is used to enhance security, to alert for falls, or to help with medication, it can be of enormous benefit to older people and their carers.

Medical technology

Managing medication for someone who needs to take a variety of pills every day is a critical task as it is important to ensure the correct dosage and timing. Modern pill dispensers can be pre-loaded with a day's, or a week's worth of medication, and will automatically dispense the right medication at the right time by sending out an alert, or sounding an alarm, to show that the medication is ready to take. Alternatively, there are medical apps where you can set reminders for when any medication is due, which medication it is and what the dosage is. You can even record that the drug has been taken and share that information with other people involved in your relative's care, such as doctors, nurses and other family members. Many conditions which require home care also require individuals to be remotely monitored, with technology enabling the recorded information to be transmitted to clinical specialists, who can offer support and intervention where necessary, based on real-time information. Search online for the relevant apps.

If an older person experiences problems due to unstable diabetes, they may be eligible for an at home glucometer. This device can record blood glucose levels and share this information automatically with their clinical team in order to create a well-informed care plan with appropriate interventions where necessary.

If someone has suffered from heart failure, they may be eligible for a heart rate and/or blood pressure monitor. This device can take heart rate and blood pressure measurements from the home and transmit them to the care team, enabling clinical staff to monitor the condition and react quickly to changes. CCGs (groups of GPs) across the country are at varying stages of implementing technology to help their patients with this. If you think it could be of benefit to your relative, speak to their GP, who can advise you if their local area already provides it.

Technology to ensure safety at home

Personal alarms are the most frequently used forms of technology for carers. They can take a number of different forms, but in essence, they allow a person to alert others when they are in need.

The most common device is one worn either around the neck or the wrist and consists of a simple push button. Pushing this button then alerts someone that the individual is in need. There are various ways in which this can be done, either via an audible alarm, which alerts someone in another room, or via a direct alert to a carer linked to a received device. This means that the carer can also wear a linked device, so that wherever they are, they can be alerted. You can also use a monitored device, which means that once the alert button is pressed, a central team is notified that a problem exists. They can then ensure that the appropriate action is taken, which could be contacting the carer, visiting the patient, or alerting the emergency services. There are also a number of apps which alert you via your smartphone.

Bed or chair sensors are the second most commonly used type of home technology device. They will alert a carer if an older person gets out of their bed or chair, or if they attempt to do so. These sensors are pads placed either on a chair, or under the sheet on a bed. When they sense that the person is attempting to stand, the carer is alerted by an audible alarm. Alternatively, if you want to be alerted specifically when a person has left their bed, you can place pressure pads on the floor by the side of the bed. When someone leaves the bed and stands on the pressure pad, the carer can be alerted.

For a relative with dementia, it can be critical to ensure that they do not leave the house unattended, or that someone is notified if they have left at an inappropriate time, or for an elongated period. You can use a device which notifies you when this happens. These alarms work by installing a sensor in the front door, which monitors when the front door is opened and closed and whenever there is movement through it. This enables a carer to be alerted immediately and to take appropriate action.

If your relative is liable to fall, the worry that they could be left alone after a fall, unable to move or stand, is constant. A fall sensor is a device worn around the neck, on the wrist or carried in a pouch. It can detect when the wearer has fallen by sensing sudden jolts, or that the wearer is not standing vertically. Once a fall has been detected, it produces an alert, in the same way as a personal alarm, to ensure that the appropriate care is provided as quickly as possible.

To check whether you might be eligible for any of the above technical support, contact your relative's GP, or your local council. You can also go online to find useful information, devices, contacts and relevant apps.

CHAPTER EIGHT

Keeping Well

As we age, it is more important than ever to keep active and well, both mentally and physically. This starts with good nutrition and taking some exercise, which includes exercising the brain.

Eating and drinking well

Eating and drinking well as we age is critical for a whole host of reasons. First, the right nutrition increases our ability to retain mental alertness, as well as helping to resist illness and disease. It also raises energy levels and improves the immune system. Eating and drinking properly also allows for faster recuperation times after illness and better management of chronic health problems, as well as helping to maintain a positive outlook on life and good emotional balance. Good nutrition keeps muscles, bones, organs and other body parts strong. Eating vitamin-rich food boosts immunity and fights illness-causing toxins. A well-balanced diet reduces the risk of heart disease, stroke, high blood pressure, type 2 diabetes, bone loss, cancer and anaemia. Key nutrients are also essential for the brain to do its job. Research shows that people who eat a selection of brightly coloured fruit, leafy vegetables and certain fish and nuts, which are packed with Omega-3 fatty acids, can improve focus and decrease their risk of Alzheimer's disease.

How many daily calories an older person needs depends on their level of activity:

- A woman over 50 who is not physically active needs about 1600 calories a day, while one who is somewhat active needs about 1800 calories a day and someone who is very active needs around 2000
- A man over 50 who is not physically active needs about 2000 calories a day, will need around 2200–2400 calories a day if somewhat active and requires 2400–2800 calories a day if very active.

Remember that every year, over the age of 40, our metabolism slows down. This means that if you continue to eat the same amount as when you were younger, you are likely to gain weight, because you are burning fewer calories. In addition, you may be less physically active.

Taste and smell senses diminish with age. Older people tend to lose sensitivity to salty and bitter tastes first, so may be inclined to salt food more heavily than before, yet they actually need less salt than the young. Try to encourage the use of herbs and olive oil to season food instead of salt, which can cause heart problems and increase the risk of stroke. Similarly, older people tend to retain the ability to distinguish sweet tastes the longest, leading some to overindulge in sugary foods and snacks. Prescription medications and illnesses can also negatively influence appetite and may also affect taste, again leading to the tendency to add too much salt or sugar to food.

Due to a slowing digestive system, we generate less saliva and stomach acid as we age, making it more difficult to process certain vitamins and minerals, such as B12, B6 and folic acid, which are necessary to maintain mental alertness, a keen memory and good circulation, so taking daily supplements is often a good idea. Loneliness and depression can also affect diet. For some, feeling down leads to not eating and in others, it may trigger over-eating. Bereavement can have a similar effect. Income can also have a major effect on healthy eating. People on limited budgets might have trouble affording a balanced, healthy diet.

However, there are a number of simple rules to follow to keep well:

- The first rule of keeping well is to drink plenty of water. As we age, we should be drinking one to two litres a day, depending on how active we are. When hydration levels are optimised, skin, eyes, energy levels and general wellbeing all benefit
- The second rule is to eat the right foods, which ensure you feel healthier. The right diet will also help skin to fight wrinkles. A diet rich in antioxidants, essential fatty acids and protein is important. It is good to eat some protein with every meal, so try to encourage your relative to incorporate meat, fish or cheese. Salmon and other oily fish provide a double bonus of helping to firm the skin and also provide plenty of healthy Omega-3. Soya, olive oil, dark chocolate, blueberries, goji berries, pomegranates, seeds, nuts, turkey and broccoli are all antioxidant rich foods and drinking antioxidant green tea, or white tea, is an excellent way of getting powerful antioxidants into your system. Eating good fats, like avocado, can help boost dry, mature skin by helping skin retain water and evening primrose oil supplements can also boost this.

Top tip: The good news is that eating a little piece of dark chocolate (the good stuff containing over 70 per cent cocoa solids) is excellent for your skin and general health. It provides the highest source of magnesium and is very high in antioxidants, which help prevent free radical cell damage. Research has also linked dark chocolate to lowering blood pressure so a small amount, once in a while, can be good for you.

Try to help your relative to enjoy food by keeping it varied. Eating a variety of different fruits and vegetables can provide many powerful nutrients and liven up meal times. Older people, especially those who live alone, can often resort to eating the same meal every day, which is boring and not as good for you as varying your diet. All major supermarkets have internet or phone delivery services, which you can order for your relative if they cannot do it for themselves. Browse with them to inspire their taste buds. There are also a number of companies who prepare meals and deliver, as well as Meals on Wheels, which you can find via your local authority, or search for them online at www.gov.uk.

Try not to overwhelm older people with large portions. Many supermarkets sell healthy kids-sized ready meals, which are perfect for the smaller appetite, easy to fit into the freezer and also low in salt and sugar. Stock the freezer and the larder with homemade meals, or ready meals if you don't have time, as well as small bran muffins and vegetables. Soups and tinned food are good staples for the larder. Make sure there is always a loaf of bread in the freezer to defrost.

Top tip: It can be a good idea to freeze several slices of bread separately, so that you do not have to defrost the whole loaf and less gets wasted.

In this way, every meal time can be easy to prepare and not too daunting, or time and energy consuming. It is also a good idea to buy healthy snacks, such as dried fruit, cereal or protein bars, mixed seeds, nuts, small juice cartons and instant soups. Frozen fruit and vegetables are an excellent way of making it very easy to access healthy ingredients, especially if mobility prevents someone from going out to buy fresh produce.

If someone has difficulty gripping standard cutlery, special cutlery is available, which makes it easier to eat. A small hot water urn may be better than a kettle as it delivers hot water in a stationary position, rather than having to lift a kettle full of boiling water, minimising the risk of scalding. Microwaves are also a quick option to prepare food.

Difficulty chewing and swallowing

Many older people find chewing difficult, particularly as their teeth deteriorate. You can make chewing easier for them by creating smoothies made with fresh fruit, yogurt and protein powder, which will also ensure they are keeping their protein levels high. It also helps to steam vegetables and eat soft food, such as couscous and rice. Yogurt and soups are also good for those who struggle to chew and swallow. Cutting food into easily swallowable cubes can help. Encourage your relative to drink plenty of water after each bite of food, as it helps with chewing and digestion and add sauces and salsas to foods to moisten them.

Preventing anorexia

Anorexia nervosa is a medical term that means lack of appetite, which sometimes occurs for psychological reasons. The condition leads to significant weight loss as a sufferer eats far less than they need to in order to maintain good health. It is a well-known eating disorder, common in teenage girls, but anorexia nervosa does occur in other age groups, particularly older people.

The cause of anorexia nervosa is not known in every instance. Although obesity can be a great cause of concern for older people, the bigger issue appears to be the decline in food intake as people age and live alone. Loss of appetite, or failure to make regular meals, leads to weight loss. This may also be caused by social or physiological factors, or a combination of both. Depression, often associated with loss or deterioration of social networks, is a common psychological problem in older people and a significant cause of loss of appetite. The reduction in food intake may also be due to reduced hunger levels. If someone is physically less active, or because older people can feel fuller quicker while eating, they tend to eat less. The central feeding drive appears to decline with age. Physical factors, such as bad teeth and ill-fitting dentures, or age-associated changes in taste and smell, may also influence food choice and limit the type and quantity of food eaten in older people.

Common medical conditions in older people, such as gastrointestinal disease, poor food absorption, acute and chronic infections and hyper-metabolism, which increases your metabolic rate can often cause anorexia, as well as deficient levels of essential nutrients and hence, poor energy. In addition, older people are major users of prescription medications, a number of which can cause malabsorption of nutrients, gastrointestinal symptoms and loss of appetite. Poor nutrition has been implicated in the development and progression of chronic diseases commonly affecting older people, with symptoms including impaired muscle function, decreased bone mass, immune dysfunction, anaemia, reduced cognitive function, poor wound healing, delayed recovery from surgery and ultimately, increased mortality. As well as weight loss, signs of anorexia include thinning hair, paleness, bluish discoloration of the fingers, dry skin, constant fatigue, dizziness and episodes of fainting, being socially withdrawn and irritability.

If you suspect that your relative is suffering from anorexia, or is losing too much weight, contact their GP. Significant or unexplained weight loss can be an indicator of a number of health problems, including cancer, so it should always be cause for concern.

Foods for arthritis sufferers

Arthritis, both rheumatoid and osteoarthritis, is an extremely painful disease, which causes joints to swell and become stiff. However, some studies have suggested that certain foods can help to alleviate the pain of arthritis. Oily fish has inflammation-fighting Omega-3 fatty acids, so try to encourage your relative to eat salmon, tuna, mackerel or herring three or four times a week. Soya also has Omega-3 fatty acids, which you can get by eating tofu or edamame beans. Cherries have an anti-inflammatory effect, as do strawberries, raspberries, blueberries and blackberries. Broccoli is high in vitamins K and C, which could help slow the progression of osteoarthritis. Wholegrains can reduce inflammation and help with rheumatoid arthritis and diabetes, so eating oatmeal, brown rice and wholegrain cereals is very helpful. Beans are high in fibre and can reduce inflammation, especially red beans, kidney beans and pinto beans. Turmeric contains curcumin and has been shown to reduce inflammation at a cellular level. Parsley also has anti-inflammatory properties and is easy to grow yourself. Eat it in salads and soups, or use it as a garnish.

Coriander helps reduce swelling and inflammation. Use it on baked potatoes, salads, soups and in Mexican and Thai food. Ginger, a staple of most Asian cookery, can soothe stomach irritation and lessen inflammation. It can be used with hot water to make a tea. It also acts as a blood thinner, so be careful with ginger if your relative is taking medicines such as Warfarin. Garlic, onions and leeks may limit cartilage-damaging enzymes in human cells and so help to prevent arthritis. Extra virgin olive oil has healthy fats and anti-inflammatory properties. Walnut oil is 10 times higher in Omega-3s than olive oil, so it is great to use on salads. Avocado and sunflower oils have proven cholesterol-lowering properties.

Citrus fruits, such as oranges, grapefruits and limes, are rich in vitamin C, which helps prevent inflammation and maintains healthy joints. Bromelain is a digestive enzyme found in the stem of pineapples, which reduces inflammation, but it should be taken in capsule or pill form. Green tea has antioxidant properties, which can help reduce inflammation. Vitamin K can also be helpful, but it can counteract blood thinners, so check with your doctor.

Exercise for older people

Please be sure to take advice from your doctor before beginning any form of exercise.

Walking

It is so important to keep moving as we age, not only to keep our bodies fit and well, but also to increase blood circulation, which benefits our brains. If nothing else, everyone should try to walk for at least 10 to 15 minutes every day. Walking keeps older people fit without the hazards of high-impact exercise and it is completely free. Older people who get about by walking are less likely to suffer mental decline, or even dementia. Brain scans revealed that older people walking between six and nine miles a week appeared to have more brain tissue in key areas. Older adults can also decrease their risk of disability and increase their likelihood of maintaining independence. Walking helps with back pain, arthritis, osteoporosis, varicose veins, reducing cholesterol and other medical problems, where inactivity is a factor and all you need is a good, comfortable pair of shoes. It also helps psychologically, by improving mood and increasing a person's sense of wellbeing through the release of endorphins.

Help your relative to work out some local walks to follow using local maps, or even initially, by driving the routes. Find local walking groups via the local authority, the library or local charities, or look online for local organised walking groups. They could even start a walking group themselves, where they plan ahead and walk to different locations from home, or as a day out. A regular morning walk with others is a great way to lift your relative's mood and give them something to get out of bed for. Maybe they can be incentivised with the thought of ending the walk with breakfast or mid-morning coffee at a local café. Or get them to borrow a dog if they do not already own one. Dogs are always eager to go for a walk, so there will be no excuse not to take them out. Walking a dog is much more fun than walking alone and dogs are great stress relievers and very good company. They alleviate loneliness as well as increasing fitness. These days you can rent a dog to walk through sites such as www.borrowmydoggy.com.

Yoga

Yoga can be very beneficial for older people. It consists of breathing exercises, relaxation and supported poses, which help improve joint mobility and flexibility, thereby reducing the incidence of falls and also pain associated with stiffness and lack of use. Weight-bearing exercise is important in maintaining bone density and strength and keeping muscles toned. Increased blood circulation affects mental alertness, as well as the physical effects of getting more oxygen to the muscles and organs, so improving their function. Breathing exercises help reduce stress, offering a sense of inner calm and mental alertness. By teaching deep breathing, more oxygen circulates around the body, bringing better health and efficiency to tissues and organs and helping to maintain a healthy blood pressure.

People who practice yoga regularly report better overall health, improved sleep and reduced reliance on medications (in consultation with their doctors). Make sure that your relative chooses a well-qualified yoga instructor, who has a good understanding of any health issues they may be suffering from, so that they can modify the practice to suit your relative's individual needs.

There are many different forms of yoga and it can be confusing. Practices like Hatha and Iyengar yoga are well suited to older people because they focus on breath control and posture, which helps to build strength and flexibility. They use props, which make the poses accessible to all. As with everything else these days, shop around until you find the teacher or class which best suits your relative's likes and needs. They can also practice yoga at home.

If you have osteoporosis, ensure that you tell the yoga teacher as certain exercises are contra-indicted (not advised).

Pilates

Eighty per cent of older people will suffer, or already suffer, with lower back pain at some time. Pilates can greatly help to relieve back pain. It is also great for strength and tone and can be an excellent stress reliever. Pilates is dedicated to improving physical and mental health, building strength from the inside and out and rebalancing the body by bringing it into correct alignment. It teaches people to understand their bodies and how they move and then shows how to apply this in everyday life.

Pilates is a series of controlled exercises, which condition the body and engage the mind. It is a balanced blend of strength and flexibility training, which improves posture, reduces stress and creates long, lean muscles without creating bulk. Pilates works several muscle groups simultaneously through smooth, continuous motion, with a particular emphasis on strengthening and stablising the abdomen, back and pelvic region (also known as the core). It acts as a bridge between physical fitness and physical therapy and can be adapted, modified and customised to meet individual needs.

Before pursuing any exercise programme, it is important that your relative checks with their doctor. Subject to medical approval, Pilates is ideal for people recovering from injury, illness, back problems, or suffering from any activity that involves repetitive movements. Pilates studios are now set up all over the country and classes are also available in many popular gyms. Classes are available at beginner, intermediate and advanced level, so there is a class for everyone. Check that class numbers are small, so that your relative can get the benefit of the instructor's attention and their advice on a personal level. Classes can also be very sociable and are a great way to meet like-minded people. They can also do one-to-one or one-to-two lessons to get personal attention from the Pilates instructor, which are very beneficial to those with specific problems, but are clearly more expensive.

Comfortable clothes should be worn to aid easy movement. Pilates is taught on mats on the floors and using a variety of specialist equipment, such as a reformer, which consists of a carriage that moves back and forth along tracks within a frame. The resistance is provided by the exerciser's body weight and by a set of springs attached to both the carriage and the platform.

If you have osteoporosis, ensure that you tell the Pilates teacher, as certain exercises are contra-indicted.

Water workouts

Swimming and aqua aerobics are very popular forms of exercise, which can be done at any age, but are particularly beneficial for older people as they are non-weight bearing. Aqua aerobics is comprised of exercises performed in shallow water, usually in a swimming pool. It typically uses the water as resistance for exercises normally done on land, such as jogging or jumping jacks. Aqua aerobics allows your relative to use water to work the heart and to strengthen and tone muscles and joints. Water buoyancy supports your weight and so the strain on joints, back and torso is greatly reduced. It is a great exercise for older people, who are increasingly likely to have had back, knee and hip surgery. Post-operatively, it can enable a speedier recovery. Stamina increases with aqua aerobics and calories can be burnt more efficiently. Due to increased resistance underwater, it burns a good amount of calories. Long-term aqua aerobics increases joint flexibility and lowers the risk of stress and anxiety, and working out in the water means no sweating and keeping cool and comfortable.

Before taking up aqua aerobics, your relative should consult their doctor, particularly if they have not been taking regular exercise before. Certain medications and old injuries may not be conducive for water aerobics. Water aerobics need to be initiated by a trained coach to avoid possible injuries. Contact your relative's local sports centre for details of the classes they run. Private health clubs also run aqua classes.

Tai Chi

Tai Chi combines deep breathing and relaxation with flowing movements. Originally developed as a martial art in 13th-century China, Tai Chi is practiced around the world as a health-promoting exercise. Studies have shown that it can help older people to reduce stress, improve posture, balance and general mobility, and increase muscle strength in the legs. Some research suggests that Tai Chi can also reduce the risk of falls among older adults and improves mobility in the ankle, hip and knee in people with rheumatoid arthritis.

Tai Chi involves proper bending and stretching of the joints by improving posture. Your relative can learn how to breathe deeply, so that they no longer have a residue of stale air at the bottom of their lungs. Tai Chi also teaches you how to move with awareness of where your weight is, so that joints are properly aligned and, over time, tendons become softer, making it easier to move the joints. Regular practice helps produce mood-enhancing endorphins in the body.

Alternative therapies

Physiotherapy

As we age, our ability to move freely can easily diminish. This can be caused by health problems or by specific injury. Physiotherapy can help to alleviate pain, improve mobility and even restore fitness in older people. It can be helpful in the treatment of back and/or neck pain, sports injuries, arthritis, heart disease, breathing problems caused by asthma or chronic obstructive pulmonary disorder (COPD), diabetes-related problems, repetitive strain injury (RSI), problems affecting the nervous system, such as Parkinson's disease or multiple sclerosis, osteoporosis, Alzheimer's disease and incontinence. Your relative may meet a physiotherapist in hospitals, or specialist clinics, and many practices will arrange home visits.

When your relative first meets the physiotherapist, they will discuss their specific problem and what caused it, and then do a physical examination to assess flexibility, strength and range of movement. Then they will devise a plan of care tailored to them as an individual. Physiotherapy is very hands-on and may include massage, hot or cold treatments, ultrasound, acupuncture, TENS (transcutaneous electrical stimulation) and hydrotherapy (water treatment). They often suggest home exercises to restore flexibility, build strength and improve coordination and balance, as well as recommending an exercise regime to help prevent future problems. They also offer advice on relevant useful aids to make moving easier, such as canes and walking aids.

Osteopathy

Osteopathy is a system of diagnosis and treatment for a wide range of medical conditions. It works with the structure and function of the body and is based on the principle that the wellbeing of an individual depends on the skeleton, muscles, ligaments and connective tissues functioning smoothly together. Osteopaths work to restore the body to a state of balance – where possible without the use of drugs or surgery – by using touch, physical manipulation, stretching and massage to increase the mobility of joints, relieve muscle tension, enhance the blood and nerve supply to tissues and help the body's own healing mechanisms. They may also provide advice on posture and exercise to aid recovery, promote health and prevent symptoms recurring. Osteopaths consider the whole person, examining posture and the strength and flexibility of muscles, ligaments and tendons.

As we age, our spines start to deteriorate and excess strain is felt through our joints and muscles. Many older people have a lower level of fitness at this stage in their lives and as a result, tend to be more prone to injury. Osteopathy treatment is designed to alleviate current problems and to help prevent reoccurrences. Nobody can reverse the effects of ageing, but osteopaths use their hands both to investigate the underlying causes of pain and to carry out treatment using a variety of manipulative techniques. These may include muscle and connective tissue stretching, rhythmic joint movements, or high-velocity thrust techniques to improve the range of movement of a joint. General releasing techniques are often used on older people to free up their movement and alleviate pain.

The plan of care is based upon the person's age, condition, lifestyle and unique spinal problem. Painkillers are not the only solution for the aches and pains associated with older age. Osteopathy can help to reduce pain and stiffness and therefore reduce an older person's reliance on medication. A good osteopath will be trained in evaluating whether a person is suitable for treatment for certain conditions, e.g. severe osteoporosis is not suitable for manipulative care.

Arthritis is suffered by many older patients. Degenerative osteoarthritis is the most common arthritis, due to wear and tear of a joint, which become painful and stiff, while rheumatoid arthritis (RA) is an inflammatory condition and harder to treat. This is mainly controlled with medication. Osteopathy cannot cure arthritis, but treatments can certainly ease pain, reduce stiffness and, hopefully, improve some joint mobility in the less acute stages of arthritis.

Older people need to keep joints loose and mobile to maintain their optimum capabilities. Osteopaths will show patients exercises that can be done daily at home to keep as fit as possible. Drinking water is very important for the joints and muscles, as older people often dehydrate without even realising it and this can lead to many illnesses, particularly urinary infections, which can cause older people to become very unwell both mentally and physically. Drinking sufficient quantities of water helps to maintain the health of joints, skin and kidneys and helps to prevent urinary tract infections, which can be extremely debilitating in older people (see pages 225–227 for further details).

Occupational therapy

Occupational therapists (OTs) aim to enable older people to make the most of their abilities to perform daily activities and to remain as independent as possible. OTs work with people who have physical and/or mental health problems in a range of healthcare settings, as well as in the community. They may work with an older person to help them keep active and able to perform their daily routines. They can teach a person with arthritis how to protect the joints and to conserve energy, help someone with a limited range of movement to do stretching exercises, use adaptive equipment and assist amputees with prosthetics. OTs can help people with poor sight to adapt their environment to avoid glare and increase colour contrast and help with memory impairment by labelling drawers and cabinets.

An OT can also assess pain and help someone to build up their stamina gradually so they can carry on with their daily activities, including scheduling activities and building in rest periods. They are expert at developing techniques to overcome pain, while remaining active and provide coping strategies, such as distraction techniques and visual imagery.

OTs also demonstrate the use of assistive equipment and technology. An occupational therapist can help with dementia, training people to help manage their daily living activities, such as bathing, dressing and eating. They encourage activities to minimise problems with memory and so help those with dementia stay at home longer. Improving environmental design helps to compensate for impaired memory and learning and reasoning skills. In addition, OTs suggest appropriate exercise or other activities, graded to an individual's capabilities to increase their quality of life, preserve their identity and provide them with a positive emotional outlet. They will also advise carers on how to support someone living with dementia.

If someone is admitted to hospital, an OT should assess them before they are discharged. This assessment will normally include agreeing goals with the patient and their carer to develop a patient-specific treatment programme aimed at achieving maximum functional ability once they leave hospital. The patient will receive a report outlining some recommendations, which may include the provision of adaptive or assistive equipment for use at home. This assistance might be provided by the hospital, your relative's local council, or may need to be purchased privately. This will depend on local policies in their area. OTs can also recommend the use of electronic assistive technology, equipment and adaptations to enable users to retain their independence, reduce care costs and remain safely at home. This work is carried out in close collaboration with district councils and NHS trusts.

OTs will advise older people and their carers on the best ways to manage at home and help retain independence for as long as possible. They focus on personal care and cooking and can even help provide some items on loan. They will advise on suitable housing and ways of adapting their home to meet older people's needs. Each council has different rules, but adaptations can be carried out on owner-occupied property and council-owned property. Housing Associations are also able to carry out adaptations to their own property. Some councils can carry out adaptations free of charge for council tenants. Older people can apply for a grant towards adapting their home to the Adult and Community Services occupational therapy service, who will conduct an assessment. Do not start adaptation work before you have had an assessment, as any financial help cannot be given in retrospect.

Reflexology

Reflexology involves the manipulation of defined pressure points on the feet, hands, lower legs, face or ears. The theory is that these pressure points correspond to various areas of the body and that the application of pressure on these specific points can help to alleviate illness, encourage healing and release tension by working on lines of energy. Reflexology is thought to be especially beneficial for older people dealing with complex and chronic conditions, such as pain, anxiety and depression, as well as for end of life palliative care. Reflexology cannot cure diseases, but it can help to alleviate the symptoms of many health problems. As a gentle, non-invasive treatment, reflexology is thought to be very beneficial in promoting a better quality of life for many older people.

Reflexologists believe that gentle massage of specific points on the feet can complement mainstream medicine, particularly by inducing a state of deep relaxation, improving blood and lymphatic circulation and helping the body's own healing processes. Regular reflexology sessions can help older people cope with general aches and pains, as well as alleviating symptoms associated with some chronic problems, including respiratory conditions, anxiety and depression, recovery from stroke, high blood pressure and migraine and headaches.

Another important aspect of reflexology is the positive impact of having one-to-one time with the therapist, of being listened to and having respectful physical contact. This can be particularly beneficial for isolated or lonely older people, either living independently, or in a care home. Reflexology for the feet is not advisable for people with foot fractures, unhealed wounds on the feet, active gout, osteoarthritis of the foot or ankle, vascular disease of the legs or feet, or thrombosis or embolism. A professional reflexologist should always be aware of foot problems which commonly occur in older people, such as sensitive skin, fragile bones, problem toenails, bunions, arthritis, reduced circulation, etc. In some cases, people can benefit from reflexology of the hands or ears instead.

After taking note of the patient's medical history, lifestyle and general health, the reflexologist will choose specific areas of the feet on which to work. Patients take off their shoes and socks and can recline in a chair, or lie on a treatment table. First, the therapist will usually start by gently massaging the feet to promote relaxation. They may use lubricating oils. Then they will apply pressure to specific areas of the feet. It is normal for this pressure to feel sensitive or uncomfortable, but it should never be painful. Some people like to have regular, ongoing weekly or fortnightly sessions. Reflexologist fees differ depending on the practitioner and the area. Reduced charges, or even free sessions, may be available from some hospitals and cancer care centres. Home visits are also possible.

Acupuncture

Acupuncture can be extremely beneficial in helping older people to restore the body's equilibrium. Traditional acupuncture is based on ancient principles dating back over 2000 years. Acupuncture views pain and illness as signs that the body is out of balance. This approach to healthcare is unique, viewing physical, emotional and mental conditions as interdependent. The treatment is based on the individual, not the specific illness, and all the symptoms are seen in relation to each other. The traditional acupuncturist's principle treatment is that illness and pain occur when the body's qi – vital energy (pronounced chi) – cannot flow freely.

Each patient is unique. Two people with the same western diagnosis may well receive very different acupuncture treatments. There can be many reasons for this, such as emotional imbalance, stress, poor nutrition, infection and injury. By inserting ultra-fine sterile needles into specific acupuncture points, a traditional acupuncturist seeks to re-establish the free flow of qi to restore balance and trigger the body's natural responses. The experience of having acupuncture is pleasant, relaxing and energising. The patient is made comfortable and draped appropriately. Needles are hair-thin, sterile and generally painless. They are never used twice. There may be a brief soreness, or pulling sensation when the needle is inserted, which means that your qi has connected with the needle. A good treatment feels like being 'in the zone' or a deep meditation as the body moves back into balance.

Acupuncture can help with depression and anxiety in the older person. In Chinese medicine, emotions are a natural part of human existence and no human being escapes being sad, angry or worried sometimes. The emotions only become causes of disease when they are particularly intense, and most of all, when they are prolonged over a long period of time, especially when they are not expressed, or acknowledged.

Acupuncture can also help to reduce over-medication in older people. No other age group is as routinely over-medicated. Combinations of medications for various ailments used in conventional medicine can exhaust and confuse the body in other ways. Acupuncture can help to balance and restore the body's vital energy flow. It offers effective pain relief. Unlike other age groups, restoring an older patient to vital health may seem to be an unachievable goal, but even a modest improvement in pain or bodily function can make a significant difference to an older person's quality of life.

Acupuncture can be very beneficial for carers. Looking after your relative can be exhausting, challenging and emotionally draining. Acupuncture can help caregivers to maintain their own life balance, restore energy and balance their emotions, so that they feel better about themselves and their quality of care

Reiki

As with other forms of complementary and alternative medicines and therapies, there is no hard scientific proof of the effectiveness of reiki. However, it does no harm and there is growing support for its use in relieving stress. As with reflexology, reiki can be particularly beneficial for older people dealing with chronic conditions, such as pain, anxiety and depression. 'Reiki' (pronounced ray-key) means 'universal life energy' in Japanese, where the therapy was first developed by Dr Mikao Usui in the early 1900s. Many Eastern medicine systems are based on the belief in a life energy which flows through all living things. Reiki uses 'hands-on healing'. There are no formal qualifications in reiki – the tradition and knowledge is passed from reiki masters on to their students.

Reiki therapists believe that they act as a channel for energy and that they can balance this energy within the body to promote a more relaxed state and an improved sense of wellbeing. Although reiki is not part of any religious practice, reiki therapists believe that it can contribute to spiritual growth. During treatment, patients remain fully clothed and can either sit on a chair, or lie down on a couch. After discussing any health issues, the reiki practitioner will move their hands on, or just above, the patient's body in a sequence of positions, which are held for two to five minutes, until the practitioner feels a change in the flow of energy. Reiki therapy can be performed on the whole body, or may be focused on a problem area. There is no massage or manipulation, and while some people report feeling some tingling or warmth during a Reiki session, others feel nothing at all. Most experience a calm feeling, however. Sometimes, there can be an emotional response.

Reiki cannot diagnose or cure diseases. However, some people have found that it can be helpful for older people coping with general aches and pains, as well as alleviating symptoms associated with some chronic problems, including anxiety and depression, migraine, headaches and recovery from surgery. Of course, for socially isolated older people, there is also an intangible benefit of having one-to-one time with the therapist, of being listened to and having respectful physical contact.

Fees for reiki treatments vary and may be available in some hospitals, NHS community services and support groups, particularly for cancer patients.

Mindfulness

Mindfulness is a therapeutic practice, where people are encouraged to be fully in the present moment. It is used as a way of managing and accepting thoughts and feelings and decreasing anxiety. The idea of mindfulness is to pay attention to your thoughts, feelings and bodily sensations calmly and without being judgemental. It is based on traditional Buddhist meditation practices, but also incorporates a variety of techniques, such as controlled breathing, as well as body awareness activities, such as Tai Chi and yoga. It can be beneficial to people of all ages and there is strong evidence to suggest that practicing mindfulness can improve people's emotional and physical wellbeing. It is used to help ease stress, depression, anxiety and chronic pain, as well as improving concentration.

Organisations such as the Mental Health Foundation promote mindfulness as an effective tool to help people improve their general wellbeing and enjoy their lives. NICE, the UK's National Institute for Health and Care Excellence, recommends mindfulness-based cognitive therapy (MBCT) for patients who suffer from recurrent depression. Cancer Research UK recommends mindfulness-based stress reduction (MBSR) as a complementary therapy to help cancer patients to cope with pain, insomnia and nausea. By relieving symptoms, MBSR helps improve the quality of patient's lives.

You do not have to be clinically depressed or ill to benefit from mindfulness. Life takes a toll on us all from time to time and older people can find it especially difficult to cope with issues, ranging from bereavement and loss of independence to new technology and an ever-changing world. Practicing mindfulness helps people resist the trap of constantly revisiting past issues and events, or getting overwhelmed by worries about the future by focusing on the present. It helps them relax, become more aware, cope with daily stress and make better decisions.

The interconnectedness of mind and body lies at the heart of mindfulness and makes it highly relevant to older people, who are more likely to experience physical health problems with associated psychological issues, such as reduced mobility and depression. It is thought that mindfulness can be particularly empowering for older people as it focuses on abilities rather than on difficulties, which may help them to feel more engaged in decisions about their care. It can also help to reduce reliance on medication and potentially help vulnerable groups in nursing homes and those with dementia.

We all practice mindfulness without thinking about it from time to time. For some people, it might be watching waves crashing onto the shore; for others it could be watching a flickering log fire, or doing a jigsaw puzzle. Whenever you are focused on the sensations of the present moment and are not carried off on a stream of anxious thoughts, you are being mindful. Practicing mindfulness usually requires a commitment of about 10 minutes to an hour each day of formal practice, sitting in a quiet place and training the mind to stop wandering and become more focused on observing the breath, relaxing the body and accepting thoughts and feelings. You can teach yourself, as there are many books and online resources available, but many older people will probably benefit from some guided sessions with an experienced teacher. There are also useful apps, such as Headspace.

Your relative can begin by practicing a few simple steps on a daily basis. They can pick a time of day to be aware of the world around them, going to the park or sitting in a different part of a room and taking note of their surroundings. They should begin to observe their own thoughts. It takes practice to put the mind in a different mode, but it is a worthwhile exercise. Or they can try meditation, where you sit silently and pay attention to the sensations of breathing, or other regions of the body. It also helps to practice yoga (see pages 119–120), where you move through a series of postures to flex the body and concentrate on your breath, or Tai Chi (see pages 122–123), where you perform a series of slow movements, concentrating on your breathing.

Pets

Pets may help older people live longer, healthier and more enjoyable lives. You have probably noticed that, when you stroke a cat, or play fetch with a dog whose tail will not stop wagging, you relax and your heart feels a little warmer. Scientists have noticed the same thing and they have started to explore the complex ways in which animals affect human emotions and physiology. The resulting studies have shown that owning and handling animals significantly benefits health – and not just for the young. Pets can ensure that older people have better physical health and mental wellbeing, stay more active, cope better with stress and have lower blood pressure. Pets need walking, feeding, watering, grooming and playing with, and so they encourage lots of playing and petting. All of these activities require some action from owners. Even if it is just getting up out of the chair to let a dog out a few times a day, or brushing a cat, any activity can benefit the cardiovascular system and help keep joints limber and flexible. Consistently performing this kind of minor exercise can help keep pet owners more able to carry out the normal activities of daily living.

Pets also help older people by providing physical contact. Many older people lack any form of physical contact from other people and renewing this through a pet has great benefits. Studies have shown that when people pet animals, their blood pressure, heart rate and temperature decrease. Pets are an excellent source of companionship, acting as a support system for older people who do not have any family or close friends nearby on a daily basis. Hence they act as a buffer against social isolation. Often older people are reluctant to go out, so they do not have a chance to see many people, but pets, particularly dogs, encourage them to leave the house and to interact. This can help combat depression, one of the most common medical problems facing the elderly. Hence, pets provide older people with a sense of purpose and a reason to get up in the morning. Pets also help them to stick to routines, such as regular times to get up in the morning, buying food and going outside, which help motivate them to eat and sleep regularly as well.

If you think that an older person might benefit from having a pet at home, talk to them before you choose one and ideally, choose with them. Make sure that they want the responsibility of a new pet, as well as the noise and the mess that may come along with it. Talk to them about whether they feel capable of feeding, watering, grooming, exercising and cleaning up after an animal. Finally, before you encourage an older person to adopt a pet, consider whether you could take care of the animal if your relative is no longer able to do so. Often, if older people reach the point where they have to leave their homes and move into assisted-living facilities, they also have to give up their pets. The number of nursing homes and other types of care accommodation that will accept animals is growing, yet still the vast majority does not allow pets. You can plan ahead and find a pet-friendly nursing facility, just in case they need to use it someday. An older person may also want to consider planning for their pet in their estate, in terms of electing a guardian and providing an allowance in their will.

Pets and older people give a great deal to each other. Research and experience has shown that animals and older people can share their time and affection, and ultimately, contribute to living full and happy lives. Though pets cannot replace human relationships for an older person, they can certainly augment them and they can fill an older person's life with years of constant, unconditional love and affection.

My father died 16 years ago and my mother was horribly lonely. Ten years ago, we persuaded her to get a dog and it has been the best decision she ever made. She loves the dog to bits and while she cannot walk her – she has a dog walker who helps her out – she has companionship all the time and someone to cuddle. So many older people never touch another person once their partner dies and animals can be an enormous source of solace.

Hobbies and activities

When your relative retires or suddenly has more spare time on their hands, there is obviously scope for them to do some of the things they have never had time to do before. Sometimes, though, it is hard to get the inspiration and the confidence to take up new hobbies and activities. There are, however, a whole host of options available. The following suggestions are by no means exhaustive, but they are hopefully helpful and thought-provoking.

Art

Art can be attempted at home, outside in the park, or in a local art class. Your relative can take up painting, drawing, sculpture or pottery. It does not matter how skilled they are as there are opportunities for everyone at all levels. The creative process is very absorbing and rewarding and it is a great way for older people to meet new people. There are also art books to help get started. Search for local art classes online.

Art appreciation

Visiting galleries is interesting and a great way to experience culture from both the past and present. There are many classes running organised trips to galleries with like-minded people to enjoy the art together, or your relative can just visit whenever they feel like it. The National Art Fund pass provides free or discounted admission to many galleries across the UK. Find out more at their website: www.artfund.org/national-art-pass.

Bird watching

You can put a bird feeder in your relative's garden and they can watch the birds eat, or they can be more adventurous and get out and about with bird watching clubs. The RSPB (www.rspb.org.uk) has all the information you need about where to go to spot the UK's favourite birds.

Bowls

Bowls is a sport for all, regardless of age, sex or physical ability, and it takes seconds to learn how to play. There are over 2500 clubs across the UK and it is a relatively cheap game to participate in compared to other sports, whether you choose to join a club, or 'pay and play' at your local park. Find out more at www.bowlsengland.com/.

Tenpin bowling

There are bowling alleys all over the UK and this is a highly social sport which is great fun. Use the safety rails until you have mastered the technique. Just search online for your local bowling alley.

Card making

Making cards is a very easy hobby to start and cards can be as simple or complicated as skills allow. It allows for creativity at all levels and is a good way to while away a few hours. It is also a great, affordable way to send good wishes to family and friends. You can buy easy card-making kits in stationers and online to get your relative started.

Cookery classes

Whether your relative is a good cook already, or new to cooking, there are cookery schools all over the country, which can introduce them to new recipes and ways to cook. They can specialise in baking, or in other specific areas or types of cuisine. Search online for local cookery courses. It is also a great way to spend fun time with the grandchildren. There are also hours of cookery demonstrations on catch up TV and YouTube.

Collecting

If your relative has something they are particularly interested in, or have a couple of things they have already collected, then building a larger collection can be very interesting and rewarding. They can go to fairs around the country, attend auctions or search online.

Computing

If your relative has never learnt how to use the internet, it is really very easy once someone shows them how and it reveals a whole new world of information and communication. They can keep in touch easily with children and grandchildren via email. Local councils run education programmes, often free of charge, or there are many private companies who offer friendly tuition. There is more information on how to get your relative connected on pages 98–103.

Dance

With the recent successful revival of dancing driven by certain well-known television shows, learning to dance is very popular. Dancing offers a great social experience and it keeps your relative fit as well. There are dance schools offering every type of dance across the UK. Just search online.

Film

Every medium- to large-sized town has at least one local cinema and new films are out all the time. The beauty of having more time on their hands is that your relative can go to see a film during the day when cinemas are quieter. Many cinemas offer cheaper tickets for pensioners and some independent groups offer season tickets. Most cinema groups offer gift vouchers, so you can treat your relative.

Flower arranging

Flower arranging courses run throughout the UK and can be very rewarding and social. Your relative can put newly acquired skills to good use at home, or impress their friends when they visit them. There are several good books which teach the basics of flower arranging, as well as demonstrations on YouTube. Search online for courses.

Golf

Golf is a very enjoyable pastime, especially if you have the time to enjoy it, as it is quite time-consuming. If mobility is an issue, most courses have buggies for hire. Most also have coaches, who are very patient with beginners and more advanced golfers alike. You can search online for your local course. There are municipal courses in most towns, which do not require membership to play, but you might want to check if you need to book a tee-off time.

Jigsaws

Traditional jigsaws are one way of keeping your relative amused and mentally alert, but it is also now possible to access jigsaws online, which means they can do a different jigsaw every day. It is a great way to while away a few hours and keeps the brain agile. Just search for online jigsaws.

Music

Music is something which almost everyone enjoys, whether it is classical, rock, pop or any other kind. Your relative can rediscover the music they enjoyed years ago on vinyl, which has made a huge comeback and basic turntables are relatively inexpensive. There are local shops selling vinyl in many towns across the UK. Or they could go to concerts, or even begin to learn an instrument, or pick up an old one they discarded years ago. Music is also very important for people with dementia and can often trigger memories which other exercises and conversation fail to do.

Photography

These days, anyone can become a budding David Bailey, whether your relative is happy to use their camera phone, or a digital camera. It can provide hours of entertainment and become quite addictive. Search online for local photography clubs, or find a course in your local area to learn the main techniques.

Reading

Reading is the biggest single pastime for older people, apart from watching television. Books provide such a wealth of entertainment, whether they are fictional, or one of the many thought-provoking non-fiction titles available, depending on your relative's interests. As people age and find very wordy books too difficult, photographic books can be very welcome and enjoyable. In addition, audiobooks are a great way for older people to still enjoy books, even when their eyesight might be failing.

Top tip: Older people might find reading on a Kindle much easier than from a traditional book because they can increase the size of the font as much as they like and the back lighting also helps legibility. They are also much lighter to hold and the touchscreen does not require as much dexterity as turning pages.

Volunteering

Volunteering can be an important way to meet new people and extend connections. Volunteers make contacts with people on a number of different levels: with other volunteers, with clients they serve and the staff of host organisations for which they volunteer. One of the other positive benefits of volunteering is that there is also scope for older people to engage in physical activities and to re-experience productive roles. Older people are viewed as a skilled, valuable, often untapped resource, possessing profound knowledge and experience, which can be utilised for a variety of worthy causes in various organisations. Some volunteer programmes for older adults try to match the skills of volunteers with appropriate opportunities and activities and this trend is becoming more common.

Volunteering is also flexible. While older people may wish to spend some of their free time undertaking voluntary activity, they may also like to spend time on other activities that they may have been unable to do while in full-time employment pre-retirement. Some people like to plan long holidays, or pursue hobbies that they were unable to devote as much time to while in employment.

Volunteering provides volunteers with a positive self-identity and sense of purpose that might otherwise be absent from their lives. This absence may be a result of the losses associated with work, primary caring responsibilities or partners and friends. Volunteering raises confidence and self-esteem and helping in the community gives people an external focus, taking attention away from their own personal concerns. Volunteering and community involvement can counteract loneliness and social isolation, as well as helping to provide mutual, functional support.

You can find more information at www.royalvoluntaryservice.org.uk.

Creative writing

Some older people enjoy writing and some even enjoy creating scrapbooks of their children and grandchildren, as well as recording their own exploits. There are also some great creative writing courses run locally or online.

Travel

Getting your relative out of the house for a few hours every so often, or every week or two is as good for them as it is for all of us. Whether you travel with them, or if they go alone, there are so many options available for older travellers.

Days out

Visiting a beautiful garden can be a very enjoyable experience for all the family. The National Trust (www.nationaltrust.org.uk) has 200 gardens and parks across England and Wales to explore. Pensioners receive 25 per cent discount off membership. The National Garden Scheme (NGS) (www.ngs.org.uk) holds events throughout the summer, many of which are free to children under 16 and pensioners. Visiting an NGS garden helps to support many nursing and caring charities. The Open

Garden Scheme provides a fantastic opportunity to see the fruits of many green-fingered amateur gardeners, who are happy to open up their gardens for the visiting public.

The UK is famous for its wealth of historic castles, stately homes, museums, art galleries and other unique attractions. Find out more via The National Trust or English Heritage (www.english-heritage.org.uk). You can also enjoy lunch or afternoon tea at most properties.

A day at the races can be great fun and tickets can be very reasonably priced. You can find the details of all race meetings at www.britishhorseracing.com.

Holidays

Including older relatives on family days out or holidays is an ideal option for some people, but it can also take some careful planning. Things to think about include journey length, accessibility of accommodation – are there accessible ramps, lifts, grab rails, etc. – activities for older people, packing medicines, assisted aids and equipment, and managing any dietary restrictions. If mobility is an issue and you are planning a UK holiday, you can check if the accommodation is compliant with the National Accessible Scheme (NAS). This helpful scheme makes it easier for you to choose appropriate holiday accommodation for your relative and for the whole family. Visit www.visitengland.com/plan-your-visit/access-all/national-accessible-scheme. There are plenty of holiday options for independent older travellers, from city breaks and package holidays to coach tours, self-catering villa holidays, river cruises and special activity holidays. You can search for a suitable destination online, or ask a travel agent or tour operator for advice and suggested itineraries.

If someone is still mobile, but does not want to travel independently, an escorted holiday might well be the answer. There are plenty of options to choose from, including coach tours in the UK, Ireland and continental Europe, as well as ocean and river cruises. If someone has more severe mobility or health issues, you may think that organising a short break or holiday is going to be too difficult, but there are specialist organisations, which offer respite care for patients and their carers. A good source of information about specialist holidays can be found at the online directory Disability Holidays Guide (www.disabilityholidaysguide.com). The national charity Revitalise (www.revitalise.org.uk) has more than 50 years' experience in helping disabled people in the UK to take essential short breaks. Options range from themed excursions and activities to respite breaks at one of their three residential centres.

Travel insurance

You will need to think carefully about the type of travel insurance an older person needs. For regular travellers, an annual travel insurance policy might make sense, although it is a good idea to check that it offers value for money and that specific medical conditions are covered. Often, single-trip policies can be a better option.

> Top tip: There are several companies offering travel insurance for older people, but it pays to shop around. Do not take the first quote offered as insurance for older people can be frighteningly expensive, particularly if they have ongoing health issues.

Available benefits and assistance schemes to help older people get around

Registering disabled

If your relative registers as disabled, their details will be stored on a confidential database and they will be given a small card as proof of registration. It does not cost any money to register. This card is a quick and easy way of proving that the holder has a significant disability and needs to use facilities provided for disabled people.

Once registered, your relative can access certain facilities when out and about, such as disabled toilets, which they can access with a key available at stations. They can also gain easier access to some concessions, such as a Disabled Persons Railcard, as well as discounts at some leisure facilities. They may be able to reclaim VAT on specific disability equipment, but all concessions are discretionary and may vary, so do check. Registering as disabled will not have any impact on your relative's applications for welfare benefits.

There are several different types of disability registration, each with their own way of registering.

Registration for people who are severely sight-impaired (blind), or sight-impaired (partially sighted)

This process does vary by area, so check with your relative's local authority first. To register, they will need to be certified as sight-impaired (partially sighted), or severely sight-impaired (blind) by a consultant ophthalmologist (eye specialist). If your relative is already attending an eye hospital or clinic, they should discuss certification with the specialist. Otherwise, ask the GP to refer your relative to a consultant ophthalmologist. If the ophthalmologist considers that they are severely sight-impaired, or sight-impaired, they will complete a certificate and send it to your relative and to their GP and to the local authority. If registered as severely sight-impaired (blind), then your relative will automatically qualify for a Blue Badge (disabled parking), blind person's tax allowance, 50 per cent reduction on TV licence fee, the London Council's Taxicard scheme (if in London) and the Disabled Person's Freedom Pass, which offers free travel in London and nationally on buses (they will also qualify for this if they are registered as just sight-impaired).

Registration for people who are hard of hearing or deaf

Please note this process does vary by area, so check with your relative's local authority first. To register, they will need to have a copy of an audiogram, which shows their level of hearing. If they have not seen an audiologist, please contact their GP for a referral to a hospital Audiology department. An audiologist can send a copy of their audiogram to the local authority, or you can do this for them. This can be sent to the social care direct team and the local authority will then send a registration card to show that your relative is either hard of hearing, or deaf with speech, or deaf without speech. If your relative is registered as deaf (with or without speech), they will qualify for a Disabled Person's Freedom Pass.

Physical disability registration

Please note this process does vary by area, so check with your relative's appropriate local authority first. To be registered as having a physical impairment, they will need to have a diagnosis of a long-term condition, which is supported by their GP. Contact social care direct, who will send your relative a form. This form must be signed to give consent for medical information to be shared with the local authority. Then you or your relative must take the form to their GP, who will complete the necessary details and return the form to the local authority. Once the local authority has received the completed form, they will issue a registration card, with either severe physical disability, appreciable physical disability (moderate), or impaired physical disability (low).

The Blue Badge

A Blue Badge will help your relative to park close to their destination, either as a passenger or driver. The badge is intended for on-street parking only. Off-street car parks, such as those provided in local authority, hospital or supermarket car parks are governed by separate rules. The badge and its concessions are for registered holders' use only and it is a criminal offence for anyone else to use the badge. Your relative can be fined up to £1000 if you use their badge without them. They must never give the badge to friends or family to allow them to have the benefit of the parking concessions, never copy the badge, or attempt to alter the details and the badge remains the property of the issuing local authority, who can ask for it to be returned if it is being misused. When using the parking concessions, the badge must be displayed on the dashboard, or fascia panel of the car, where it can be clearly read through the front windscreen and if there is no dashboard or fascia panel in the vehicle, they must still display the badge in a place where it can be clearly read from outside the vehicle. The front of the badge should face upwards, showing the wheelchair symbol. The side showing the photograph should not be visible through the windscreen. The details on the front of the badge must remain legible and if they become unreadable through fading or wear and tear, the badge must be returned to the local authority to be replaced.

Blind people need to ensure that people displaying the badge or clock on their behalf understand how to display them correctly. The clock should be received together with the Blue Badge. Incorrect display of the badge may result in a parking fine. They must display the blue clock when parked on yellow lines, or in other places where there is a time restriction. The blue parking clock must show the quarter-hour period of arrival. It should be displayed on the vehicle's dashboard, or fascia panel, so that the time can be seen clearly through the front windscreen.

Top tip: Don't assume that your relative's Blue Badge works in all areas of the region where they live or throughout the UK. My mother used hers in one borough of London, but not the one where she had registered, and received a parking ticket. Clearly, this is not the most well-thought-out scheme as it assumes disabled users will not travel out of their area!

Your relative can now apply or renew a Blue Badge online if they are resident in England, Scotland or Wales, and you can apply on behalf of the applicant. They will first be asked to identify their local authority and provide some personal details to help the local authority deal quickly with their application. This will include their National Insurance number, driving licence number, if they have a driving licence, and their Blue Badge number, expiry date and the name of the issuing local authority, if they have one. They will also need to provide a passport-style photograph as this will appear on the back of the badge. The photograph will not be on display when the badge is used in the vehicle. The photograph can be submitted with the online application, if they have a digital photograph that can be uploaded. Alternatively, they can send a signed photograph to their local authority.

At the end of the application form, your relative will be notified of what they need to do next. This may include sending in proof of address and identity. They will be asked for details of their medical condition and the difficulties they have when operating parking meters. If they drive an adapted vehicle, they will be asked to provide a photocopy of their insurance details to verify the adaptation. Any information that they supply will be transmitted securely via the government's internet to the local authority that is responsible for issuing Blue Badges in the area where they live. The information will only be able to be accessed by the local authority processing the application. A limited amount of information will be accessed by enforcement officers to prevent abuse of the Blue Badge scheme.

Your relative must return the badge securely to their local authority if the badge has expired, or their medical condition or mobility improves so that they are no longer eligible. More details are available at www.gov.uk/apply-blue-badge.

Transport concessions and assistance

Buses

Older and disabled people are entitled to a minimum concession of free off-peak travel on a local bus anywhere in England. Off-peak times are between 9.30 a.m. and 11 p.m. on working days and all day at weekends and public holidays. Concessionary bus travel is available at other times. If your relative was born before 6 April, 1950, they are eligible for an older person's bus pass from their 60th birthday. Women born after 5 April, 1950 become eligible for an older person's bus pass when they reach pensionable age. Men born after 5 April, 1950 become eligible when they reach the pensionable age of a woman born on the same day. For more details on eligibility, see www.gov.uk. Some services are not covered by this provision, such as coaches, shuttle buses to special events, tourist services or services on vehicles of historical interest, e.g. open-top tours, rail replacement services and services where extra provision, such as refreshments or car parking, are included in the fare.

Some local authorities may offer further concessions to their residents – for example, concessions on trams or rail travel, or travel during peak hours – but these will only apply in the specified local authority area. Where local authorities offer more generous schemes, they are allowed to make a charge for a bus pass as long as a free bus pass providing the statutory minimum concession remains available as an option. All modern buses should be wheelchair-accessible and are also easier for people who have difficulties in walking, climbing steps or holding handrails as they have level access or lower entry and exit steps and easier-to-grip handrails.

Trains

The Senior Railcard is available to anyone (including visitors to Britain) aged 60 or over. It costs £30 for one year, or £70 for three years (prices change so please check online, or at your local station) and allows your relative to save one-third of the cost of most rail fares in Great Britain. There may be other offers for cardholders, such as reduced-price membership for art or food societies. It is available from railway stations, or from rail-appointed travel agents. To apply, take the completed form and proof of age, such as passport, driving licence or birth certificate, to the nearest staffed railway station, or to a rail-appointed travel agent. Your relative can also purchase a Senior Railcard online.

The Disabled Persons Railcard costs £20 for a year (or £54 for three years) – prices do change, so please check online or at your local station – and it allows your relative to save one-third of the cost of most rail fares in Great Britain. If you are travelling as a companion, you are entitled to the same reduced rate. There are also discounts for people who travel in their own wheelchair, or those who are registered blind, or partially sighted. People who need to stay in their own wheelchair during a journey and do not hold the Disabled Persons Railcard can still get discounts on single and return tickets. They can get the same discounts for one travelling companion. Registered blind and partially-sighted people who do not have a Disabled Persons Railcard can also get discounts, but only if they travel with a companion. They must show a document confirming their disability when they buy a ticket or when travelling. Train companies can provide special arrangements for disabled or mobility-impaired passengers. For example, your relative may be able to arrange for staff to help get on and off the train, or when changing trains. Contact the train company as far in advance as possible and at least 24 hours before the journey.

For people with hearing and speech impairment, stations normally display printed timetables. Many ticket office windows have been fitted with induction loops to help hearing-aid users. Most stations display arrival and departure details on visual display units. For people who are visually impaired, train arrivals and departures are usually announced over loudspeakers. Many stations have toilets that are accessible to wheelchair users and convenient for other disabled travellers. Some toilets for disabled passengers are kept locked to deter vandalism and a notice will indicate where a key can be obtained. Some toilets are fitted with National Key Scheme locks. Facilities on trains also vary. Newer trains are designed to allow full access for people with disabilities, including people in wheelchairs, but older trains may be less accessible.

Coaches

There is no national concessionary coach scheme. Facilities for disabled people vary between coach stations and companies and your relative should check with their travel agent, or the coach company, regarding what facilities are available at both ends of the journey and along the way. Many coaches are not accessible to some disabled people, because they have steps. Most cannot carry wheelchair passengers, unless the coach has been specially adapted, or the passenger is able to sit in a normal coach seat and their wheelchair can be folded and stowed in the luggage lockers. Many coach operators will provide assistance for disabled people, although seven days' notice is usually required so the arrangements can be made.

Planes

Some airlines may offer concessions for older people, but the qualifying age may be different for different airlines, so do check. For details of any concessions that may be offered for a particular journey and the qualifying conditions, contact a travel agent, or the airline. Contact the airline and/or the airport before your relative travels to find out what facilities are available for people with disabilities or mobility issues at the airport and on the plane and whether any particular arrangements for assistance need to be made. Make sure you let the airline know of your relative's needs at least 48 hours before flying.

Ships and ferries

Some ferry companies offer discounts to Senior Railcard holders and others may offer discounts to passengers above a certain age. Check with the travel agent, or the ferry company, to see what discounts may be available. Facilities for people with disabilities vary both at terminals and on board.

Community transport options

If your relative is disabled and cannot use ordinary public transport and does not have access to a car, there are community transport schemes that they may be able to use. To get information on all community transport resource available in their area, you can use the map provided on the Community Association or from the local authority. Search for your local Community Association online. There are also schemes where people volunteer to use their own cars to drive those who cannot use public transport. They can take your relative to visit a doctor, chemist, or to go shopping, or even to social events, or to visit friends or family. In some areas, the local Royal Voluntary Service (RVS) provides social car schemes (www.royalvoluntaryservice.org.uk). Local branches of the British Red Cross www.redcross.org.uk or St John Ambulance (www.sja.org.uk) may also run voluntary schemes, so it is worth checking online.

Dial-a-Ride schemes provide door-to-door transport for people who cannot use public transport. They use converted cars or wheelchair-accessible minibuses with fully trained staff. Most Dial-a-Rides will only take your relative on local trips. Usually, you have to book their trips in advance and enrol as a member. There may be a call-out charge, and they will probably have to pay a mileage cost. Check for your local service online.

Taxicard schemes have been set up on a local basis by some local authorities. They are for disabled people who cannot use the bus service due to difficulties with access. The schemes offer a number of concessionary taxi journeys each year. Contact the local council to find out whether it runs such a scheme and what concessionary fares it offers.

Shopmobility schemes lend manual and powered wheelchairs and powered scooters to those people who need them to shop and use other facilities in town centres. There are schemes running throughout the UK. Check online.

Transport for London free travel for over-60s

If your relative lives in London and is aged 60 or over, you can apply for a 60+ London Oyster photocard to travel free on bus, Tube, tram, DLR, London Overground and most National Rail services in London. To apply online, they need a colour digital photograph, an active email address, a machine-readable passport (most valid travel passports are machine-readable), or a UK driving licence (full or provisional), a valid debit or credit card (registered to their current address), payment of the £10 admin fee and verification of their address (www.tfl.gov.uk/fares-and-payments/adult-discounts-and-concessions/60-london-oyster). Your relative can get a Freedom Pass if their only, or main home, is in a London borough and they were 60 or older before 6 April, 2010, or if they turned 60 on or after 6 April, 2010 and meet the new age criteria, or have an eligible disability. You can find more information at www.londoncouncils.gov.uk/services/freedom-pass/older-persons-freedom-pass.

CHAPTER NINE

Medical Matters

This chapter does not seek to answer all your medical questions and is not written by doctors, but it will provide you with an overview of the main physical and mental problems which affect us all as we age and provide information on where to seek further help.

The important regular check-ups everyone should have

If your relative takes the time to undergo some basic routine health check-ups regularly, it is so much easier to spot problems in the early stages and get treatment sooner rather than later.

Eye tests

An eye test checks vision, but just as importantly, it can detect signs of a number of other conditions, such as diabetes, often before your relative has any symptoms. An optometrist examines your relative's eyes for any evidence of abnormality, injury or disease and will ask them to read letters from a chart. They will also test eye pressure by directing a puff of air at the eye to calculate the pressure inside and check for glaucoma. After the test, the optician will tell your relative if they need any sight correction and if so, they will usually help them with that at the time. If there are any signs of further eye complications, the optician will refer them to their GP, or to an eye specialist. Over the age of 60, your relative is entitled to a free NHS sight test every two years and, if aged 70+, they may be entitled to a free test annually.

Hearing tests

Hearing tests are crucial, as many people suffer from deficient hearing as they age and this can lead not only to difficulties following conversations, but also to isolation and dementia. Following a conversation about any hearing difficulties, an audiologist will examine your relative's ears with a light called an auriscope, which is a small torch with a magnifying glass, which allows them to see into the eardrum. They will check for any discharge coming from the ear and check the eardrum for bulging eardrum, which means there is infected fluid in the middle ear; for dull eardrum, which means there is uninfected fluid in the middle ear (this is known as glue ear); for retracted eardrum, which means the Eustachian tube is not working properly; for perforated eardrum, which means there is a hole in the eardrum, which may or may not be infected, or for foreign bodies which might be blocking the ear, including ear wax. The Eustachian tube is a narrow passage leading from the pharynx to the cavity of the middle ear, permitting the equalisation of pressure on each side of the eardrum.

The audiologist may then carry out simple tests using their voice to determine the extent of any hearing loss. These might include pure tone audiometry (PTA), where a machine (audiometer) produces sounds at different volumes and frequencies (pitches). Your relative listens through headphones and responds when they hear them by pressing a button. There is also a speech perception test, which tests the ability to hear words without using visual stimulus. Words are played through headphones, or spoken by the tester. Tympanometry tests can confirm whether there is any fluid behind the eardrum and if the Eustachian tube is working normally. A small plastic bung seals the ear and the machine changes the ear canal pressure. The whispered voice test involves the tester blocking one of the ears and testing your relative's hearing by whispering words at varying volumes. Your relative will be asked to repeat the words as they hear them. The tuning fork test measures different aspects of hearing. The tester taps the tuning fork on their elbow or knee to make it vibrate and then places it in different areas around your relative's head. It can determine if your relative has conductive hearing loss, caused by sounds passing freely into the inner ear, or sensory-neural hearing loss, where the inner ear is not working properly. The bone conduction test involves placing a vibrating probe against the mastoid bone behind the ear and measuring how well your relative hears sounds transmitted through the bone. It is a more sophisticated version of the tuning fork test and can check if hearing loss is emanating from the outer and middle ear, the inner ear, or both.

The type of hearing loss your relative has is important, because it determines what help or treatment is most suitable. The audiologist will then recommend hearing aids, or refer them to a specialist. Your relative should get their hearing checked annually and tests are usually free. However, if you need financial help with the cost of hearing aids, you must contact your local authority, or the NHS.

Dental checks

It is very important to have regular dental check-ups. Not only can teeth have decay, but gums can as well. Infection in the gums can lead to infection in the bloodstream, which can cause other, more serious problems, and if gums erode, it is much harder to fix than actual teeth. If any work is necessary, the dentist will explain the next steps. The dentist will also take a medical history, including the use of anti-psychotic drugs, anti-epileptics, antidepressants, beta-blockers, and diuretics, which can all cause a reduced saliva production. Poor saliva production makes it much harder for denture wearers and there is a higher risk of tooth decay and gum disease in people with dry mouth, due to the lack of cleansing effect from the saliva.

Older people are more vulnerable to tooth decay, sometimes because of a preference for sweeter foods, or taking less care with their oral hygiene and inability or reticence to access dental treatment. The dentist will check heavily filled teeth, or teeth under crowns and bridges. They may look sound, but the nerves in these teeth may die off and then the dead nerve tissue can become infected and toothache can follow. The dentist will also look for broken teeth, which can leave sharp ends and result in tongue ulceration.

Checking for gum disease is critical, as it causes bone loss, tooth loosening, or even tooth loss and requires treatment. Ninety per cent of gum diseases can be prevented by effective oral hygiene, so regular tooth brushing is essential and using an electric toothbrush is preferable. It also helps to floss regularly and to have check-ups with the hygienist. The dentist will also look for any lumps, white lines and patches. Your relative should get their teeth checked every six months. They may be eligible for free dental treatment, but you have to contact your local NHS dentist to discuss eligibility

Bowel cancer screening

Bowel cancer screening can detect potential problems, even when people have no symptoms. The testing kit, called a fecal occult blood test (FOBT), is posted to your relative and they then collect stool samples on a special card, which are sent to a laboratory for analysis. Bowel cancer is the third most common cancer in the UK. Eight out of 10 people who get cancer of the bowel are over the age of 60. Screening is offered every two years to all men and women aged between 60 and 70. The test looks for blood in the stool and if there is any, your relative will be asked to repeat the test. Their GP may then recommend a bowel examination (colonoscopy) to rule out cancer. About 2 per cent of people will have an abnormal result and will need follow-up tests.

Cervical screening

Cervical screening aims to detect cervical abnormalities. Cervical cancer is the 11th most common cancer in women. Early detection and treatment prevents up to 75 per cent of cancers developing. A doctor or nurse inserts an instrument known as a speculum to open the vagina and uses a spatula to sweep the cervix to take a sample.

It is a slightly uncomfortable procedure. Women aged between 25 and 64 are eligible for a free cervical screening test every three to five years. Results should come back within six weeks. An abnormal result requires further investigation and treatment.

Prostate test

While there is no national screening programme for prostate cancer, it is worth getting a check done – which is just a simple blood test – through your relative's GP, as it can prove a lifesaver. Symptoms may include needing to go to the toilet more often and difficulty passing urine, as well as blood in the urine or semen. Be aware that many men suffer from some of these symptoms from having an enlarged prostate gland, which is actually a benign condition. Making sure that it is benign rather than cancerous can provide peace of mind, as well as helping to prevent a serious condition from worsening. It is worth getting a regular prostate test over the age of 50 anyway, as early detection has a very high cure rate. It is a simple blood test and not invasive at all.

Cholesterol test

Cholesterol is a type of fat that is carried by the blood around the body. High levels of cholesterol can clog the arteries and increase your relative's risk of a heart attack or stroke. High cholesterol does not cause any symptoms, so the only way to find out is to take the test. Cholesterol is measured with a simple blood test by the GP and should be checked annually. If your relative has high cholesterol, they can make some simple changes to their diet and exercise regime. Their doctor will help them and may refer them to a dietician. The GP may recommend statins in certain cases, which are a group of medicines that can help lower the level of low-density lipoprotein (LDL) cholesterol in the blood. This is often referred to as 'bad cholesterol'. Statins reduce the production of it inside the liver. There can be side effects from taking statins, so ensure that you discuss these with the doctor.

Blood pressure tests

High blood pressure can weaken the heart and damage arteries, increasing the risk of heart disease, stroke and kidney disease. In the UK, about 50 per cent of people over 65 have high blood pressure, but many do not realise it. The GP will place a cuff around the upper arm and inflate it until it becomes tight. The test is quick and painless. A blood pressure reading below 130/80mmHg is normal. The first/top number refers to the amount of pressure in your arteries during the contraction of your heart muscle. This is called systolic pressure. The second/bottom number refers to your blood pressure when your heart muscle is between beats. This is called diastolic pressure. If results are abnormal, your relative will need to have their blood pressure checked regularly. If it is consistently high, they may need to make lifestyle changes, including eating more healthily and taking exercise, and possibly have to take medication. Get them to get it checked annually. It is free at their GP's surgery.

Breast screening

Breast screening (known as a mammogram) detects breast cancer early. A third of breast cancers are now diagnosed through screening. Each breast is placed alternately on the X-ray machine and is compressed with a clear plate. It only lasts a few seconds, but it can be slightly uncomfortable. The result will be sent to your relative within a fortnight. If the result is abnormal, they will be asked to go for further tests, such as an ultrasound or needle test. Women are invited for a mammogram between their 50th and 53rd birthdays and then every three years until they reach the age of 70. After the age of 70, they can request a mammogram every three years.

Skin checks

Keeping an eye on moles can help your relative to spot the early signs of skin cancer. Most moles are harmless, but they can develop into skin cancer (known as malignant melanoma). Deaths from melanoma have tripled in the last 30 years for people over 65. Skin cancer is linked to sun exposure over a lifetime, so older people are more likely to develop the disease. If your relative notices a strange mole, ask their GP to look at it. If the GP is concerned, they will refer them to a specialist for further testing. Your relative should look out for a change in colour, size or shape of existing moles and check moles regularly themselves, or ask someone else to do so if they are on their back. They can take a photograph and then compare it with a more recent photograph to help see if anything has changed.

Overview of medical conditions affecting older people

Arthritis

The term arthritis literally means 'joint inflammation', but it is generally used to refer to more than 100 different conditions, which affect the joints and may also affect the muscles and other tissues. Osteoarthritis is the most common form of arthritis, which happens due to the breakdown of the tissue inside the joints. Rheumatoid arthritis is an autoimmune disease. This is when your immune system, which usually fights infection, attacks the cells that line your joints, making them swollen, stiff and painful. Despite the prevalence of the disease, the causes are not completely understood.

There is no cure for arthritis and many different factors may play a role. Incidences of osteoarthritis increase with age due to simple 'wear and tear' on the joints – the older you are, the more you have used your joints. However, it is not an inevitable part of getting older, because not everyone suffers from it. Increased body weight adds stress to lower body joints and is a well-established factor in the development of osteoarthritis. The knees carry the brunt of someone's body weight and are particularly at risk.

Top tip: Keep your weight down. Did you know that every extra pound a person gains adds four pounds of pressure on the knees and six times the pressure on the hips? Gaining weight increases the likelihood of developing osteoarthritis and therefore the likelihood of needing hip and knee replacements, so it helps to keep any excess weight off.

Athletes and people whose jobs require repetitive motion (such as landscaping, typing or operating machinery) have a higher risk of developing osteoarthritis, due to injury and increased repetitive stress on certain joints. Soft tissue injuries can also lead to osteoarthritis, which can also appear in joints affected by previous bone fractures and surgeries.

Genetics play a role in the development and progression of osteoarthritis, particularly in the hands. Inherited bone abnormalities affect joint shape or stability, or defects that cause cartilage to form abnormally. It is also more common in joints that do not fit together smoothly, such as those of people who are bow-legged or double-jointed, but having these traits does not necessarily mean osteoarthritis will develop. Studies show that weakness of the muscles surrounding the knee is associated with osteoarthritis, especially in women, and makes the pain and stiffness worse after onset. Strengthening exercises for thigh muscles are important in reducing the risk.

One of the main symptoms of osteoarthritis is its effect on the cartilage of a person's joints. Cartilage acts as a cushion or hinge in between the joints. When everything is working well, the cartilage protects the bones of the joint from rubbing together. In someone with osteoarthritis, the cartilage around the affected joints begins to wear away. This, in turn, causes the bones in the joint to begin to rub directly against one another, which can be incredibly painful. It is also common for this to result in small bone fragments breaking away, which can cause infection and disability. In the body, any joint can fall victim to the effects of osteoarthritis, but it is most often found in the hips and knees, which are weight-bearing. It can also be found in smaller joints, such as the hand. In most cases, only one joint in a pair will be affected by this disease; for example, in someone with knee osteoarthritis, if the right knee were infected, the left knee would typically not be affected. This is referred to as an asymmetrical arthritis. Sufferers will generally have pain, swelling or stiffness in one or more joints, or in the back or neck or after heavy activity, such as gardening or housework, after long walks, or when getting up in the morning.

Rheumatoid arthritis is classified as an autoimmune disorder, which means that it causes the body's own immune system to attack itself. The immune system is used to fight infection, but in someone with rheumatoid arthritis, the body thinks that the joint is actually an infection. As a result, the cells in the body begin to attack and break down the joint, causing rheumatoid arthritis. The exact trigger of this autoimmune disorder is not known. Rheumatoid arthritis shares a number of similarities with osteoarthritis, but it is considered to be symmetrical arthritis, i.e. usually joints are affected uniformly. Sufferers experience stiffness, throbbing and aching pain, which is often worse in the mornings and while resting, rather than after activity. As the lining of the affected joint becomes inflamed, it can cause the joints to swell and become hot and tender to touch. The condition can also cause inflammation of the tear glands, salivary glands, the lining of your heart and lungs, and your blood vessels.

There is no cure for arthritis, but there are many ways to make life more comfortable and to keep mobile and independent:

- Try to keep weight down to avoid unnecessary wear on the joints
- Keep a good balance of adequate rest with sensible exercise (such as walking, cycling and swimming), but stop any exercise or activity that increases the pain
- Arthritis responds better to warm conditions, so a hot water bottle, warm bath, electric blanket or microwave-heated wrap can soothe the pain and stiffness
- Try to avoid getting too cold
- Physiotherapy and osteopathy can be helpful in improving muscle tone, reducing stiffness and maintaining mobility
- Shoe inserts (orthotics), good footwear and a walking stick can help painful knees, hips and feet
- Aspirin, ibuprofen and paracetamol can all be effective painkillers, but the doctor may prescribe special anti-arthritic medication if required, or may refer your relative to a pain specialist to consider cortisone injections
- There is a wide range of inexpensive equipment and tools that can help with cooking, cleaning and other household chores. These can be discussed with the doctor, physiotherapist, or occupational therapist.

Surgery can be considered to relieve severe pain for most joints. The new techniques and artificial joints are improving all the time. Replacement of a worn-out hip joint with an artificial hip made of a combination of metal, or plastic, is a very common operation and can be done as keyhole surgery in most cases. More than 90 per cent of these are successful. Modern knee replacements are also giving excellent results, and if your relative has crippling knee pain, this operation can bring great relief.

You can find more helpful information at Arthritis Care (www.arthritiscare.org.uk).

Bladder

The bladder and bowels are two important organs. They are at the end of the digestion process and work to filter out what the body does not need or want. Looking after these organs is essential, because in doing so, your relative can avoid urinary and fecal incontinence. The smallest of lifestyle changes and choices can have a positive, immediate impact on the bladder and bowel.

People who have issues with a weak bladder, or occasional urge incontinence, will often assume that, to control it, they need to control their fluid intake. Unfortunately, this can make incontinence worse, especially if your relative has an overactive bladder or urge incontinence. The bladder, when dehydrated, will become more irritated and the condition will appear worse. As counterintuitive as it sounds, encourage your relative to drink plenty of water, slowly increasing their intake to about two litres a day. Glugging a pint of cold water is not the best way to solve incontinence either. Most health professionals recommend spreading drinks throughout the day, but to try to have most fluid intake by 6 p.m. to help manage nocturnal toilet visits.

Caffeine and alcohol are stimulants on the bladder and can contribute to inflammation and further irritation. Both also have a diuretic effect on the body, so when your relative drinks these, they need the toilet more often. Carbonated drinks can also make them urinate more and caffeine is not just found in ordinary tea and coffee, so check food labels carefully. Many people find that by drastically reducing or cutting out caffeine altogether, their overactive bladder is much more manageable. Sadly for many, avoiding chocolate bars and hot chocolate drinks can also be helpful in controlling the symptoms of an irritated bladder.

Fruit juices are acidic and although we may think of them as healthy, they can be a major cause of an irritated bladder. Encourage your relative to keep fruits and juices to a minimum. Hot or highly spiced foods can also be a major cause of bladder irritation, because they stimulate the body, so ask your relative to consider cutting out, or decreasing their intake of spiced foods, including chilli peppers and salted fish and meats, as well as instant soups, noodles and some stock cubes and gravies. Some diet or low-fat products contain artificial sweeteners called aspartame and saccharin, two known bladder irritants, so sugar-free drinks or low-fat yogurt may also cause a few bladder issues.

You can find more information at Bladder & Bowel Community (www.bladderandbowel.org).

Bowel

Bowel cancer can affect any part of the colon, rectum or anus, which are the three main parts of the large bowel. It usually starts as slow-growing polyps or ulcers attached to the inside of the bowel wall. These can gradually start to change and become abnormal over time. Untreated, these polyps and ulcers can gradually increase in size, becoming cancerous. There are many common conditions that can affect the health of our bowels. Many symptoms are similar to those of bowel cancer, so it is important to get your relative checked out by their doctor. The doctor will examine them and take a careful history to make sure that whatever is causing the problem is investigated properly and treated promptly. Your relative should not be embarrassed, or put off, as it is so important to get any possible problems checked out. Bowel cancer claims a life every half an hour and it affects men and women almost equally.

The good news is that bowel cancer can be successfully treated in over 90 per cent of cases, if it is diagnosed at an early stage, before it has had a chance to grow and spread. Regular bowel cancer screening has been shown to be very effective in detecting early changes in the bowel. Bowel cancer screening aims to detect signs of bowel cancer at an early stage before obvious symptoms occur. It is available to eligible people every two years and everyone eligible is urged to take it up when offered. Screening kits are sent through the post automatically, to the address registered with the GP. In England and Northern Ireland, screening is offered to people between the ages of 60 and 69, although in England, this is gradually being extended to include people aged between 70 and 74. In Scotland, people are currently offered screening from ages 50 to 74, and in Wales, they are offered screening from ages 60 to 74.

If your relative is over the eligible age for automatic screening, they can still request to be sent a screening kit by calling the bowel cancer screening helpline free on 0800 707 60 60. The existing screening programme is a simple FOBT (fecal occult blood test), which detects blood hidden in the small samples of poo. The test is completed at home over the course of a few days and then returned by post to a central laboratory for testing. It involves handling faeces, so although the test is simple, some people may be a bit squeamish. The test does not diagnose bowel cancer, but can find blood in the poo. A positive test will trigger an invitation to retake the test. If this is also positive, the patient will have further investigations (a colonoscopy, where a camera is inserted into the bowel) to find out what is causing the bleeding.

We all experience problems with our bottoms and bowels from time to time. Usually there is nothing to worry about. However, if your relative notices certain symptoms for more than three weeks, then they must see their GP. The early symptoms for bowel cancer can include blood in faeces, or loose stools for three weeks or more, although these are very similar to other, much less serious problems with the bowel. It is very important to be aware of what is normal, so they can recognise any unusual changes and act quickly to get them investigated. Chances are that it is nothing to worry about, but these symptoms could be signs of bowel cancer, so get your relative to tell their doctor. Finding bowel cancer early makes it more treatable and could save their life. Your relative must see their doctor if they have rectal bleeding without any obvious reason, especially if it is unusual and does not respond to prescribed treatment for more common problems, such as haemorrhoids.

A persistent change in bowel habit, especially if they are going to the toilet more often, or experiencing unexplained looser stools, should also be checked. Symptoms may also include unexpected constipation and a feeling of fullness in the rectum for three or more weeks. Constant, unexplained pain anywhere in the abdomen, especially if it is severe, is also of concern. It may also be linked to going to the toilet, or it might come and go, like cramps or colic. Check out any unexpected lump in the stomach, especially if it is on the right-hand side, unexpected weight loss, perhaps due to lost appetite, or feeling bloated or sick or unexplained tiredness, which is a symptom of anaemia. Most people with these symptoms do not have bowel cancer, but the GP will want to examine your relative and may do further tests to rule it out. While the exact causes of bowel cancer are unknown, there are certain things that can be done to reduce the risk of developing it – for example, getting more exercise, eating a better diet or reducing alcohol intake, or stopping smoking.

Symptoms could be caused by other common conditions that can easily be treated and managed. Piles or haemorrhoids are soft swellings just inside the anus, often accompanied by other symptoms, such as pain and itching. They can cause bright red bleeding from the bottom and you might be able to feel them with a finger, especially after going to the toilet. Anal fissures, which are tears in the skin around the opening of the anus, are often caused by constipation. Irritable bowel syndrome (IBS) is a collection of symptoms, such as stomach cramps or pain, diarrhoea and/or constipation and a change in bowel habits caused by inflammation and infection in the lining of the bowel. People with IBS do not have higher risk of developing bowel cancer, or any other serious bowel condition. Crohn's disease, diverticular disease and ulcerative colitis are other common inflammatory bowel diseases with symptoms that include abdominal pain, tiredness, weight loss, sores, bloating, bleeding and mucus. These diseases can also put you more at risk of developing bowel cancer and the GP should monitor this regularly.

You can find more information at Bowel Cancer UK (www.bowelcanceruk.org.uk).

Dental problems

Older people are more vulnerable to tooth decay, possibly due to a preference for sweeter foods, less care with their oral hygiene, weakening enamel and inability or reticence to access dental treatment. Tooth decay is largely preventable by reducing the quantity and frequency that sugar is consumed. If you eat five times a day and brush with fluoride toothpaste at least twice a day, it is hard to develop tooth decay. Remember, even fresh fruit eaten in excessive amounts causes tooth decay. Food grazing throughout the day is especially bad, as it means that there is sugar and acid against the teeth all day. Rinsing with water will help to dilute any sugar or acid (in the case of fruit) and then the application of fluoride toothpaste as a tooth 'ointment' can prevent further tooth decay.

Heavily filled teeth, or teeth under crowns and bridges, may look sound, but the nerves in these teeth may die off. Once this happens, the dead nerve tissue may become infected and toothache can follow. The ideal treatment would be root canal treatment, or possibly extraction. If it is not possible to get to a dentist, a combination of painkillers (ideally, ibuprofen) and antibiotics can be used if prescribed by a doctor. Antibiotics normally take a minimum of 24 hours to work, so it is important to control any pain with painkillers. Always read the instructions and try to take them regularly and especially before bed, when pain can be particularly severe.

Decayed teeth, worn teeth and old fillings do break, often leaving sharp ends that the tongue plays with. This can result in tongue ulceration, which can be very sore. Ideally, your relative should ask the dentist to smooth off the sharp piece as soon as possible or they might need a filling replacing or removing. Gingivitis (bleeding gums) is present in almost all mouths and is not especially significant, but should be checked out if it persists. Gum disease can cause bone loss, tooth loosening, or even tooth loss. A dental check-up is the opportunity to assess the level of gum disease. Ninety per cent of gum diseases can be prevented by effective oral hygiene, which should include cleaning in between the teeth with small brushes or dental floss. There is no evidence to suggest that mouth rinses make a significant difference, but an electric toothbrush can be more effective than a manual brush. Food impaction can cause sore gums. Small brushes or flossing will prevent this.

It is not uncommon to see a range of lumps, white lines and patches in the mouth. Ulcers are common, but, if they have not healed within two weeks and there is no obvious cause (sharp tooth or filling), the ulcer should be investigated by a dentist. Any lump or patch in the mouth should be investigated if it bleeds or changes in size, appearance or ulcerates. Mouth cancers account for over 2 per cent of all cancers and their incidence is increasing. Smokers are at increased risk and if the person has a history of smoking and heavy drinking, the risk of oral cancer increases by 16 times.

Old age itself can eventually lead to a reduction in saliva gland function, but anti-psychotic drugs, anti-epileptics, anti-depressants, beta-blockers, and diuretics can all cause a reduced saliva production. Poor saliva production makes it much harder for denture wearers and there is a higher risk of tooth decay and gum disease in people with dry mouth, due to the lack of cleansing effect from the saliva. Using sugar-free gum and regular sips of cold water can help and there are saliva substitute sprays available. Increased toothpaste use is important to prevent tooth decay. Diabetics are more vulnerable to gum infections. People with dementia must be individually assessed for dental problems. Most dental treatments are done without anaesthetic or with a local anaesthetic, but some conditions may require a general anaesthetic and this may only be available in a hospital.

Prevention is the easiest cure. Regular dental check-ups, liberal use of fluoride toothpastes and effective oral hygiene twice a day should be encouraged.

Dentures

Dentures are removable false teeth, which replace original teeth, if they have become sufficiently damaged. They are made from either metal or acrylic. While the aim is always to keep your own teeth, some people, even those who have looked after their teeth, may need dentures at some point as they age. Obviously, if your relative does lose teeth, it can affect their ability to eat, speak properly and may affect their self-confidence too. Dentures can also enable them to continue to eat well, speak properly and feel that they have the self-confidence to face the world. Depending on your relative's dental problems, they may need either complete or partial dentures. Their dentist will advise on the best solution.

Dentures are made by the dentist, who will take an impression from your relative's mouth. This is done by placing a tray with dental putty inside, which is pushed around the teeth and gums and takes an impression of the mouth and its specific shape. Those impressions are then sent to a dental technician to be custom-made. The dentist will match the shape and colour of the dentures as far as possible to your relative's natural teeth. If some of their own natural teeth are still in good condition, they may only need partial dentures. These are usually a metal or plastic plate, to which a number of false teeth are attached. This plate is then either fastened by means of a metal clasp to your relative's natural teeth, which can be removed, or alternatively, the dentist may place crowns over some of the natural teeth to anchor the partial denture.

There are several types of complete dentures. There are complete immediate dentures (also called full dentures), required if all your relative's teeth need to be removed. Usually these dentures can be used immediately after the extraction of any remaining natural teeth, so that your relative does not have to manage without any teeth at all. Complete immediate dentures fit over the gums and jawbone. However, gums and bone may shrink, especially during the first six months after teeth extraction as part of the gums' natural healing process. If this happens, your relative may have to have their dentures adjusted to ensure they still fit well. Complete conventional dentures are required if the gums need to heal before your relative can wear dentures. While they may have to manage without teeth for a few months, when they finally get dentures, they should fit well and not require further adjustment, as the gums will have already shrunk.

An implant is a good option if your relative has suffered too much bone loss for conventional dentures, or is unsuited to them. Between four to six implants are placed within each arch of the mouth, which contain special fittings, to which the dentures will attach. This requires the creation of a hole through the gum into the jawbone, where the dentist will insert an artificial titanium root. These titanium roots require between two to six months to fuse with the bone, after which time the dentures can be attached. Implants help to preserve the amount of remaining jawbone, which is crucial for supporting the dentures. Your relative might be advised to wear their new dentures all the time until they get used to them and after that, they will normally take them out when they go to bed, depending on the type of dentures they have. Implanted dentures are not removable. It is worth noting that dental implants help to preserve the amount of jawbone which forms the foundation to support the denture.

For NHS dental patients in England, dentures cost £256.50, coming under Band C of dental charges. Prices are subject to change, so do check on the NHS website. If you have dentures fitted privately, partial dentures will cost anything from £500 and complete dentures upwards of £2,500. The cost of implanted dentures depends very much on how much work your relative needs, but they can expect to pay anything from £3,000 upwards. Ask their dentist for a written quote before proceeding.

Your relative should clean their dentures just as they would clean their natural teeth – often and well. If they are removable dentures, it is best to brush them with toothpaste and/or soap and water to remove food and dental fixative before soaking them in denture cleaning solution. They should try not to drop them, as they can crack and break. If they take their dentures out at night, they should put them in water so they do not warp. If they have dental implants, they can clean them just as they would clean their natural teeth. Well cared-for dentures may last years, but they will need to be checked regularly. They may also need to be relined from time to time, which is a method of adjusting the internal part of the base of the dentures with an acrylic resin to correct their fit. If your relative's dentures feel as if they are fitting badly, ask their dentist to check them immediately, as badly fitting dentures can give severe discomfort and may lead to mouth sores and infections. Eventually, their dentures will probably have to be made again due to changes in their mouth and gum shape over time. Some people who have been wearing full dentures over long periods can find it difficult to have well-fitted dentures made.

When someone starts to wear dentures, it can be a good idea to begin eating soft food, but once they have got used to them, they should be able to eat as they did before. While your relative is getting familiar with their dentures, they may want to use a fixative to help keep them in place. This may also be the case if the gums have shrunk. However, tight-fitting dentures should not require any adhesive to keep them in place.

Dental anxiety

Dental anxiety – a fear of dentists – is very common. It affects one in every six adults in the UK alone. If your relative is afraid of the dentist, then it is much better to find a sympathetic one. In particular, you want to find a dentist who will work with your relative to help them to become less anxious and one who is prepared to take treatments and check-ups slowly to give them as much time as possible to prepare mentally and put them at ease as much as possible. Many dentists will offer an initial meeting without any invasive procedures. This is a great way to get to know them and see if they will be a good fit for your relative. Before you choose a practice, read some reviews online to check how the dental practitioners are reviewed. In order to overcome dental anxiety, your relative needs to be able to share their problems with their dentist and others. Sharing dental anxiety with the dentist is essential, but sharing with friends and family is also a great way to get some additional support and help.

Top tip: Controlled breathing is a very useful technique which helps to relax the body and gives your relative something to focus on during dental treatment. Simply breathe in through the nose for an internal count of three, and then exhale for a count of three. Repeat this and focus the attention on maintaining a steady, rhythmic breathing pattern. This helps reduce stress and distracts the patient from their mouth.

Dental prevention is better than cure

If you want to make the dentist as pain-free and relaxed as possible for your relative, then they need to keep their oral hygiene levels very high. You want to make sure that they are brushing at least twice a day (preferably three times) and flossing regularly. This will help to destroy plaque and keep gums healthy, which are just as critical as the teeth. If you can encourage your relative to perfect their oral hygiene routine and spend time every day working on their teeth, they will be able to avoid 90 per cent of all the most common oral problems. In addition, it helps to cut down on sugary food and they could try chewing gum to reduce plaque and keep the mouth as healthy as possible.

Diabetes

Diabetes is a condition where the amount of glucose in the blood is too high, because the body cannot use it properly. This is because the pancreas does not produce any insulin – or not enough – to help glucose enter the body's cells, or the insulin that is produced does not work properly (known as insulin resistance). Insulin is the hormone produced by the pancreas that allows glucose to enter the body's cells, where it is used as vital fuel for energy, so we can work, play and generally live our lives. Glucose comes from digesting carbohydrate and is also produced by the liver. Carbohydrate comes from many different kinds of food and drink, including starchy foods, such as bread, potatoes and chapattis, fruit, some dairy products, sugar and other sweet foods. If your relative has diabetes, their body cannot make proper use of this glucose, so it builds up in the blood and is not able to be used as fuel.

There are two types of diabetes – type 1 and type 2.

Type 1 diabetes develops when the body's immune system attacks and destroys the cells that produce insulin. As a result, the body is unable to produce insulin and this leads to increased blood glucose levels, which in turn can cause serious damage to all organ systems in the body. Nobody knows for certain why these insulin-producing cells have been destroyed, but the most likely cause is the body having an abnormal reaction to the cells. This may be triggered by a virus, or other infection. Type 1 diabetes can develop at any age, but usually appears either before the age of 40, or especially in childhood. Type

1 diabetes accounts for between 5 and 15 per cent of all people with diabetes and is treated by daily insulin injections, a healthy diet and regular physical activity.

Type 2 diabetes develops when the body does not produce enough insulin to maintain a normal blood glucose level, or when the body is unable to use the insulin that is being produced effectively. Type 2 diabetes usually appears in people over the age of 40, although it can appear earlier in Southern Asian and black people, who are at greater risk. It is also becoming increasingly more common in children, adolescents and young people of all ethnicities. It can also be caused by being overweight. Type 2 diabetes accounts for 85 to 95 per cent of all people with diabetes and is treated with a healthy diet and increased physical activity. In addition to this, medication and/or insulin are often required. Type 2 is reversible if the correct diet and exercise regimes are implemented and maintained.

Diabetes is a common condition that can have a significant impact on the health and wellbeing of older people. The medication that is required to control the condition may be more likely to cause side effects, because of changes in the circulation and kidneys as people get older. Becoming diabetic in later life can complicate existing health problems, such as arthritis, heart trouble and memory problems and may be catastrophic for a vulnerable older person.

It is not always easy for your relative to eat well when they have diabetes, but one of the most important rules is to eat regularly, so do not let them skip meals and remind them that breakfast is the most important meal of the day. So, after a night of fasting, make sure they start the day off with a healthy breakfast in order to get their metabolism firing. As far as possible, try to encourage your relative to space meals evenly throughout the day. If there is a possibility that they may miss a meal, such as going on a long journey, or having a day out, remind them to take a small meal with them as back-up, such as a salad or a sandwich.

They must also remain hydrated, ideally by drinking 8 to 10 glasses of fluid per day. Water is by far the best refreshment for diabetics, but milk, tea and coffee, and herbal teas work, as do citrus fruits, such as oranges, although citrus fruit may be too acidic for some older people. It is important for us all to carry a small bottle of water during warmer weather, but this is particularly important for diabetics. Sugary drinks should be avoided as much as possible, but do not necessarily have to be cut out altogether. Hot drinks should ideally be drunk without sugar, or with artificial sweeteners. Take advice from a dietician.

It is very easy to eat too much and many older people are of a generation that always makes sure they leave a clean plate no matter how much food is put on it. Portion size is a very important issue in supporting healthy eating for diabetics, as weight control is crucial.

The best ways to reduce over-eating include:

- Drinking plenty of water with meals to fill up and be less tempted to take second helpings
- Using smaller plates so it is difficult to put too much food on them
- Putting healthy vegetables on the plate first with a main meal to fill the plate up and leaving less room for the fattier stuff. It will fill you up more as well.

Fats are essential to a healthy diet and everybody needs them, but there are good and bad fats. Saturated fats are the ones which should be avoided by all of us, but especially by diabetics, and although many manufacturers have cut down on saturated fats in their foods, they are still found in many everyday foods, such as cakes, processed meats, butter and cheese, so check the ingredients when shopping for food. It is better to avoid ready-made meals and processed foods.

Carbohydrates are an important part of any diet. Healthier wholegrain starchy foods, fruits and vegetables, pulses and some dairy foods are all good sources of carbs. But all carbs affect blood glucose levels. As a diabetic, your relative will need to be particularly conscious of the amount they eat to control their blood sugar levels. If they need specific guidance on the type and amount of food they should be eating, speak to their GP or to a dietician.

Too much salt contributes to high blood pressure and this can cause complications for diabetics in particular, so should be avoided. As people age, their sense of taste diminishes and so they will often add more salt to their meals when cooking and at the table. Adults should not have more than one teaspoon (5g) of salt per day. Cooking from fresh ingredients will help keep salt levels low and reduce the risk of high blood pressure.

Top tip: Removing the salt cellar from the table can be a very simple way to help reduce salt intake, as is adding herbs and spices instead.

Encourage your relative to include fish in their diet as much as possible, as it is an excellent form of protein. It does not matter if it is fresh, frozen or canned – it is still good for you as long as there is no added salt. Fish fried in batter is best avoided, but if it is too tempting, your relative can always just pick out the fish inside and leave the batter. Oily fish, such as mackerel and salmon, is rich in Omega-3, protects the heart and helps with brain power, as well as being a good food for diabetics, so stocking up your relative's larder with cans of oily fish is a good idea – they are easy to serve, soft to eat and very healthy.

Eating five portions of fruit or vegetables a day is really crucial for a good diet in order to get the range of vitamins, minerals and fibre needed. For any older person, sometimes the best way to eat their five a day can be by drinking it. There are many types of machines available which can liquidise fruit and vegetables into tasty drinks for an older person and these can even be made into batches and frozen. Just be careful about how much salt and sugar is contained in the fruits. Choosing seasonal produce will help to keep down costs too.

Some sugar can be eaten by diabetics, but really only in moderation. It is best to consider something sugary as an occasional indulgent treat. Artificial sweeteners should be used when sweetening food and drink whenever possible. It is also very tempting to buy foods labelled as 'diabetic', but they really do not offer any real benefit to diabetics and indeed may do harm, as they may still affect blood glucose levels. They are often expensive and contain as much fat and calories as ordinary versions. Once again, fresh unprocessed items are always going to be healthier.

More information is available at Diabetes UK (www.diabetes.org.uk).

Eye problems

There are several eye problems that become more common among people as they get older, although they can potentially affect anyone at any age.

The cornea and eyelids

The cornea is the clear, dome-shaped window at the front of the eye. It helps to focus light that enters the eye. Disease, infection, injury, and exposure to toxic agents can damage the cornea causing pain, redness, watery eyes, reduced vision, or a halo effect. Treatments include making adjustments to the glasses prescriptions, using medicated eye drops, or having surgery.

The eyelids protect the eye, distribute tears, and limit the amount of light entering the eye. Pain, itching, and tearing are common symptoms of eyelid problems. Other problems may include drooping eyelids, blinking spasms, or inflamed outer edges of the eyelids near the eyelashes. Eyelid problems can often be treated with medication or surgery.

Presbyopia/long-sightedness

Long-sightedness is the loss of the ability to see close objects or small print without glasses clearly. It is a normal process that happens slowly over a lifetime. Presbyopia is often corrected with reading glasses or bifocals. Your relative can try ready-made reading glasses, which can be bought from most pharmacies or supermarkets. Start with a low-level lens, such as a +0.5, or +1, and increase it gradually if needed, or your relative should visit an optometrist for an eye test and bespoke glasses. Be careful with bifocals when you or a relative first wear them, as it takes a while for the brain to get used to them and they can cause dizziness and even falls.

Everyone over the age of 40 should have a two-yearly eye examination, even if they do not need glasses, just to check the health of the eyes. Most people find they cannot read without reading glasses once they have read with them, as their vision is much clearer and there is less strain on the eyes.

Floaters

Floaters are tiny spots or specks that float across the field of vision. Most people notice them in well-lit rooms, or outdoors on a bright day. Floaters are often normal, but they can sometimes indicate a more serious eye problem, such as retinal detachment, especially if they are accompanied by light flashes. If your relative notices a sudden change in the type, number of spots or flashes they see, they should visit the GP as soon as possible, who will refer them to an ophthalmologist.

Dry eyes

Dry eyes happen when tear glands cannot make enough tears, or produce poor-quality tears. Tear quantity and quality reduces with age and many people, particularly women, get dry eyes. Symptoms are gritty, itchy, red and burning eyes and the eyes may even water as the body tries to flush away the irritation with 'reflex' floods of tears as there is not enough continuous 'background tear' production. You can try lubricant drops or gels from the pharmacist, or have them prescribed by the GP. If neither helps, your GP or optician may suggest that your relative tries a humidifier at home, or uses humidifying aerosols. The GP might also suggest preservative-free drops, or drops with hyaluronic acid. Tear duct plugs or surgery may be needed in more serious cases of dry eyes, but results can be variable.

Too many tears

Having too many tears can come from being sensitive to light, wind, or temperature changes. Protecting the eyes by shielding them or wearing sunglasses can sometimes solve the problem. Tearing may also mean that your relative may have a more serious problem, such as an eye infection, or a blocked tear duct. They should see their GP or optician in the first instance, who can refer them for treatment for both of these conditions. The cause may be excess tear production, poor-quality tears (see above), or blepharitis, which is inflammation of the eyelid margins. If eyelid margins are crusty, sticky or red, blepharitis is usually the culprit. It can be improved by keeping the lashes clean by bathing them with dilute baby shampoo, or blepharitis solution and cotton wool balls daily. There are also eye wipes available, which should be used twice daily. Heated eye bags can also be very effective. It is also worth trying Carbomer gel four times a day for a month to see if reflex tearing is the problem. If this does not work, then see your optometrist or GP. If the eyelid is lax, or the tear duct blocked, referral to an ophthalmic surgeon for further expert advice and treatment may be appropriate.

Top tip: I struggled with blepharitis for years, which caused many painful corneal ulcers. I now use a hot microwaveable eye bag for 10 minutes each evening and bathe my eyes morning and night with Optrex eyewash and Blephaclean eye wipes. I use Viscotears gel at night. It's a boring routine, but my eyes have never been better!

Conjunctivitis

Conjunctivitis is a condition in which the tissue that lines the eyelids and covers the eyeball becomes inflamed. Sometimes called pink eye, it can cause redness, itching, burning, tearing, or a feeling of something in the eye. Conjunctivitis occurs in people of all ages and may be caused by infection, exposure to chemicals and irritants, or allergies. This can be treated by buying chloramphenicol drops over the counter at the chemist. Once opened, they should be kept in the fridge and discarded after one month. Be careful about sharing towels with someone with conjunctivitis, as it is highly infectious.

Cataracts

Cataracts are cloudy areas that cover part of, or the entire lens, inside the eye. From middle age onwards, the lens gradually becomes cloudy and this is cataract formation, but the speed of this formation and how much it affects vision varies. Cataracts often form slowly, without pain, redness, or tearing in the eye. Some stay small and do not alter eyesight. In a healthy eye, the lens is clear like a camera lens and light has no problem passing through it to the back of the eye to the retina, where images are processed. When a cataract is present, the light cannot get through the lens as easily and, as a result, vision can be impaired. Symptoms include glare in bright sunlight and headlights, and blurred vision, particularly in the distance when reading road signs and recognising people from a distance. If they become large or thick, cataracts can usually be removed by surgery. If your relative develops symptoms, they should see their GP. If they are diagnosed with cataracts, it is probably reasonable to go for surgery. Cataract surgery and replacement of the lens with an implant is high-tech, but very safe these days. It is usually done under local anaesthetic, so age is not a barrier. HM the Queen has just had hers corrected at the age of 92 and carried on with a royal wedding and the races straight afterwards! Patients of 100 years old are commonly treated and more than 95 per cent of them will have an improvement in their vision with no complications. However, if your relative feels that they can see well even if they have some cataract, there is usually no need to consider an operation until they find there is more of a problem with their sight. The operation is the same whether the cataract is mild or more severe, so your relative can wait until they feel they need it.

Glaucoma

Glaucoma develops when there is too much fluid pressure inside the eye. Glaucoma affects one in 50 people over the age of 40 and this incidence increases with age, so it is relatively common. It is a disease of the optic nerve that causes insidious painless damage to sight. The eye pressure is usually, but not always, elevated. Holes in the vision at the side occur, but these are only noticed when the disease is very advanced. There is no treatment that will cure loss of vision, so it needs to be prevented. As most people are unaware that they suffer from glaucoma, everyone over 40 years should see an optometrist every two years for an eye examination, even if you do not need glasses. The optometrist will check the eye pressure with a puff of air, do a visual field test and look at the optic nerve. If any of these tests are abnormal, your relative may be recalled for a repeat test, or referred to an eye clinic. Treatment is usually prescription eye drops, but occasionally laser or surgery. Glaucoma treatment is usually needed for life. Note: glaucoma runs in families, so if your relatives or grand-relatives suffered from it, you are at greater risk.

AMD

Age-related macular degeneration (AMD) damages the middle of the retina and causes difficulty reading right up to total loss of central vision and being unable to recognise friends and family. It is the most common cause of visual loss in the UK and your relative's risk is increased by smoking. It comes in two forms. The first form is dry AMD, where the central retina becomes worn out with age and reading and then distance vision is gradually lost. There is no specific treatment for dry AMD, but a good bright light and magnifying aids may help. A minority of people progress to the second more severe form – wet

AMD – in which abnormal blood vessels grow and leak under the retina. This causes distortion of vision, so that straight lines appear to have a bend in the middle and central vision is blurred. If your relative notices this, they should see their optometrist as soon as possible and will be referred to their local eye hospital for further tests and treatment. Note there are many vitamin supplements sold, but these have only been medically proven to be effective for people who have intermediate, or wet AMD, not mild dry AMD, and the tablets need to contain the AREDS formula, so check the box. (The original AREDS formulation contains vitamin C, vitamin E, beta-carotene, zinc and copper. In 2013, NEI reported the results of the follow-up study, called AREDS2. The AREDS2 formula studied vitamin C, vitamin E, copper, lutein, zeaxanthin, omega-3 fatty acids and a lower amount of zinc.)

Top tip: Anyone noticing sudden loss of vision in one eye should never ignore it. Phone the optometrist immediately and ask to be seen that day. If your relative cannot see an optometrist, they should get an emergency appointment with the GP, or go to A&E. They will need to be examined and then it can be decided how urgently they need to be seen by a specialist. If loss of vision is gradual, make an appointment to see an optometrist, not the GP, as they have the best training and equipment to assess you.

The NHS has further information on eye care for the over-60s. Visit www.nhs.uk/live-well/healthy-body/eye-health-tips-for-older-people.

Falls

Falls are common in older people and the risk of falling increases with age. A third of those aged 65 years and over, rising to over 40 per cent of those aged 80 years and above, fall each year, compared with 8 per cent in middle age. A fall may be the result of a simple trip due to an environmental hazard, such as poor footwear, wet and slippery floors, loose rugs or poor lighting, but often it is caused by additional factors affecting the person themselves.

Physiological changes associated with normal older people reduce balance, increase reflex times and thus, increase the risk of falling. Specifically, we rely on our vision, sensation from the feet and legs, the inner ear and processing of all these inputs by our brain. Even in healthy old age, all of these systems show physiological decline, putting us more at risk. Additionally, without regular exercise or training, we lose muscle strength and blood pressure control on changing position (e.g. standing up) becomes less effective, which may cause unsteadiness and dizziness. Chronic problems, such as osteoarthritis, eye disease and inner ear problems are also often present and increase the risk of falling. Acute problems, such as infection, heart rhythm disturbances and drug problems, can also cause a fall or loss of consciousness. Thus, falls may be caused by a single factor, but much more commonly by a combination of environmental, physiological and pathological factors in older people. Neurological problems, such as dementia, can cause metabolic disturbance, as do certain drugs or drug withdrawal (including alcohol), environmental change, strokes, Parkinson's disease, loss of sensation, particularly in feet and disc disease or spinal osteoarthritis. Falls can also be caused by vertigo.

Many drugs are capable of increasing the risk of falling, but only a careful medical history will help establish if this is likely. You should read patient leaflets carefully and ask the GP if any new drug or combinations of drugs may increase the risk of your relative falling.Drugs can cause falls due to lowering of blood pressure, particularly when standing, or by causing drowsiness and increasing reflex times. They can also slow the heart rate and cause low blood sugar. Visual defects, such as cataracts, macular degeneration and glaucoma, can also contribute to falls, as can arthritis and foot problems. Disuse of muscles leading to wasting and weakness can also cause falls.

Homes should be checked for poor lighting, loose rugs and carpets and uneven steps. Footwear should have good grip and walking aids should be appropriate (see pages 78–83 for tips on ensuring good home safety).

Falls can have serious consequences, including head and soft tissue injuries, as well as fractures. A fear of further falls can limit an older person's activities and unchecked, can lead to isolation, further physical decline, depression and even institutionalisation. A lengthy lie on the floor, if someone is unable to get up by themselves, can potentially lead to muscle breakdown and kidney damage, pressure sores, hypothermia and the effects of missed medication. Two-thirds of all falls in older people lead to hospitalisation, which brings its own complications.

If an older person falls, do not ignore it. Consider making an appointment with the GP, who will assess risk factors, give advice and may refer your relative to a falls service in hospital. If an underlying medical condition is found, a drug review may be necessary. A strength and balance programme through the physiotherapy service may be offered and a care assessment to optimise independence and safety at home (see pages 70–73 for details on the care assessment). Bone health should be assessed, so that osteoporosis can be detected and treated, resulting in a lower chance of fracturing a bone in a fall. This may require answering some questions, but in some cases may warrant a bone-density scan. Everyone, regardless of whether or not they have fallen, will benefit from regular exercise, as this will increase mobility and balance (see pages 118–123 for suggestions). You may want to consider a fall alarm for your relative.

The NHS has further information on falls at www.nhs.uk/conditions/falls.

Gout

Gout is the most common form of inflammatory arthritis and occurs when crystals of sodium urate form inside joints. Typically, it presents with sudden, severe pain in the joint, together with redness and swelling. Gout attacks can last between three and 10 days. Gout is a chronic progressive condition and can develop in any joint, but it seems commonly to affect the big toe joint. There is a separate condition known as pseudo gout, which is caused by crystals of calcium pyrophosphate forming in the joints.

The cause of gout is an excessive build-up of a usually harmless chemical called uric acid (urate) in the blood. Urate is made in the body every day and results from the breakdown of chemicals called purines. It is usually filtered out by the kidneys and excreted in urine. When too much uric acid is produced, or not enough is excreted from the body, uric acid builds up and can cause tiny, gritty crystals of sodium urate to form in the joints and this leads to inflammation.

Top tip: An enduring myth about gout is that only older men can get it. Certainly, gout is most common in men aged 30 and over, but it can affect people of all ages. Gout actually affects 1 in 7 older men and 1 in 16 older women. This makes it the most common type of arthritis after osteoarthritis.

According to the charity Arthritis Care, gout affects 1 in 40 people in the UK and since 1997, there has been a 30 per cent increase in patients diagnosed with gout. Furthermore, this figure is increasing by almost 2 per cent every year. While more men than women get gout, the risk for women increases after the menopause as the body produces less oestrogen, which facilitates the excretion of uric acid. Risk factors for gout include high blood pressure, genetic predisposition (close relatives with gout), chronic kidney problems, a diet rich in purines (found in foods such as sardines and liver), sugar-sweetened soft drinks, fruit and fruit juices with high levels of fructose and drinking too much beer, wine or spirits.

It is important to get proper medical treatment for gout, as it can lead to long-term health problems, including joint damage, kidney stones, and cardiovascular disease. Most people take anti-inflammatory painkillers to cope with gout attacks. A key treatment for gout is known as urate-lowering therapy (ULT), which aims to lower uric acid levels sufficiently to prevent new crystals forming and helps to dissolve existing crystals. This is done with drugs, such as Allopurinol or Febuxostat. ULT can eventually lead to a permanent elimination of sodium urate crystals and a 'cure' for gout. However, patients normally have to continue the treatment daily to maintain the effects. Getting appropriate medical advice and treatment is essential, but there are also some simple diet and lifestyle changes which you can make to prevent gout attacks. Losing weight can help to lower uric acid levels in the blood and tends to improve general health. A calorie-controlled, sensible diet plan is recommended. Regular exercise reduces urate levels and will therefore decrease the risk of developing gout (for more details on exercise see pages 118–123). It also makes people feel more energised and healthier. It is a good idea to drink less alcohol, especially beer, stout and port wines, as these are known to raise the level of uric acid in the blood.

Some foods contain very high levels of purine, which can raise uric acid levels. Foods to avoid include offal (liver and kidneys), game (rabbit, pheasant), oily fish (sardines, mackerel, anchovies), seafood (mussels, crab, shrimp), and foods high in yeast and meat extracts such as Marmite, Bovril, and commercial gravy. The best foods to eat include fruit, vegetables, starchy carbohydrates (potatoes, bread, pasta, and rice) and some milk and dairy. Soft drinks sweetened with sugar are known to increase significantly the levels of uric acid in the blood, so avoid drinking these. Consumption of fruit juices high in fructose should also be reduced. Staying hydrated is important and will help to reduce the amount of uric acid in the blood, so drink plenty of water, ideally up to two litres per day. There is evidence that vitamin C (500mg per day) can reduce the risk of developing gout. It is thought that vitamin C increases the amount of uric acid excreted in the urine.

Top tip: Get regular blood pressure checks. People with gout tend to have higher blood pressure, so it is a good idea to have regular checks at least once a year. Contact your GP's surgery.

Arthritis Research has further information on gout at www.arthritiscare.org.uk.

Hearing loss

There are various types of hearing loss, which can affect each and every one of us at some point regardless of age. Hearing loss can stem from various sources including noise, traumas, medication and hereditary conditions. The most common case of hearing loss is age-related, however. Early signs of this type of hearing loss can appear from the age of 40, but it is far more evident in the over-60s. It is associated with the overall decline of the human body and the detrimental effects of the increased number of free radicals which damage cells, including those responsible for hearing.

Our inner ear contains tiny hair cells tasked with capturing vibrations in the air (what we refer to as 'sound'). Once captured, these are sent to the brain by way of the hearing nerve. As the body matures, their number and quality diminishes, resulting in a growing difficulty to hear certain sounds. Hearing loss can also be noise-induced. Our contemporary lifestyle means that we are exposed to man-made sounds, some at a level which have a devastating effect on hearing ability. Exposure to harmful sounds over short or long durations can cause irreversible damage to the inner ear parts. Thankfully, unlike age-related hearing loss, using noise protection and distancing yourself from the source of the sound can help reduce the likelihood of noise-related hearing loss. Some people may also suffer temporary hearing loss due to infections, such as common flu. These are usually treatable using medication.

The severity of the symptoms of hearing loss may vary from one person to the next. They can include difficulty in hearing the people around you within noisy environments, where background noise may seem far too loud compared to the actual speech, and sound generally seems less clear.

Your relative may not be able to hear the telephone or doorbell ring when others can, other people may sound mumbled or slurred, and they may have an inability to hear high-pitched sounds such as 's' and 'th'. This could lead them to have to ask people to repeat themselves, or to have the television or radio turned up much higher than other family members. Hearing loss can also make older people feel tired after participating in a conversation held within background noise.

Unfortunately, age-related hearing loss is an irreversible condition. Inner ear hair cells cannot regrow or regenerate. Recommended treatment revolves around managing the condition. There are medical devices which can help overcome hearing impairment, but equally, those around a hard-of-hearing person can help by demonstrating their support. Family members, caregivers and partners can try to ensure that the cause of the hearing loss is understood to be an issue. When engaging in a conversion with someone who struggles to hear, attempt to position yourself facing the person so that they are able to read your lips. In addition, speaking clearly in a normal manner is essential as shouting can cause distortion of sound. Most importantly, be patient and do not allow yourself to become frustrated. It is just as frustrating for the person trying to hear and demonstrating empathy can be very constructive.

There are plenty of devices designed to help the hard-of-hearing to overcome hearing loss on a daily basis. The most common are digital hearing aids, which are small devices that fit inside or outside the ear and help amplify external sound. Other devices which fall under the category of assistive hearing devices include amplified phones, doorbells, loud alarm clocks and induction loops. Hearing aids and assistive hearing devices do not cure hearing loss, but they do make it possible to carry out many daily activities without relying on external help. Any hearing-loss management solution should follow a hearing test taken at a reputable hearing centre.

Top tip: Did you know that hearing aids take patience to use and manage? Often older people hear whistles and distortion and struggle to get the volume level right. Also, the batteries are very small and fiddly, which is not user-friendly for older, arthritic hands. So be patient.

There is an association between hearing impairment and dementia, but there is little evidence to suggest that a hearing impairment alone leads to a decline in brain function. One study found that 50 per cent of people with a mild hearing loss and dementia improved when hearing aids were fitted. They found that hearing aids did not improve their cognitive function, or reduce behavioural or psychiatric symptoms, but it did show that patients improved because they could hear better and engage with others more easily.

The NHS has more information on dealing with hearing loss at www.nhs.uk/conditions/hearing-loss.

The heart

Blood pressure

Controlling your relative's blood pressure is important, as if the pressure is too high, it can make them vulnerable to heart attack and stroke. Blood pressure is represented by two numbers, which show the highest and lowest pressure the blood exerts during the heartbeat cycle.

Systolic pressure is the highest force the blood exerts against the arteries when the heart contracts and diastolic pressure is the lowest force the blood exerts while the heart is resting between contractions. Ideally, blood pressure should be 120/80 or less. If it is higher than this, but below 140/90, then it is still considered normal, but cardiovascular risk increases and you should try to lower it. Discuss diet and exercise options with your GP, as well as possible medical help. Blood pressure is considered too high if it runs consistently over 140/90. Low blood pressure is usually measured at 90/60 or less, but unless you often feel faint or dizzy, it is usually nothing to worry about. Some conditions, such as diabetes and Parkinson's, can also lead to low blood pressure, as can certain medications your relative might be taking for other conditions.

High blood pressure puts people at risk of developing cardiovascular disease, as it puts the heart under strain and damages the interior linings of the arteries, which makes it easier for layers of fatty cholesterol to build up. If there is a short-term increase in blood pressure when stressed, this can cause blood clots, which can lead to a stroke or heart attack. It is therefore very important not only to have a healthy resting blood pressure, but also good blood pressure control during times of emotional and physical stress.

There are medicines available to help control blood pressure, but your relative can also make lifestyle changes which will help. Being overweight and having a large waist measurement and a high waist girth can increase blood pressure. Try to encourage your relative to reduce excess weight with exercise and by maintaining a healthy diet. Too much alcohol can also raise blood pressure, so make sure they are careful and do not binge drink. Exercise makes the heart work more efficiently and this helps regulate blood pressure. Just half an hour a day of activity will help, but check with your relative's doctor before they start any exercise programme, if they have not done any for a while. If their blood pressure is consistently over 140/90, then they should consult their doctor for further advice.

Your relative should stop smoking, as it raises blood pressure with the very first drag, due to the effect of the nicotine. Smoking also damages the walls of the arteries, which makes your relative more susceptible to high blood pressure in the future. Salt can mean that they retain fluid in the blood, which can increase blood pressure. Many ready meals and other pre-prepared food contain a great deal of salt, so try not to add more.

Top tip: Bananas contain potassium, which is good for the heart, as well as providing a great energy boost.

Stress drives blood pressure up, so encourage your relative to manage it through exercise, sleep and relaxation techniques, such as mindfulness (see pages 131–133 for more details).

Managing cholesterol

Cholesterol is a fatty substance which is found in the blood. Mainly made in the body, it plays an essential role in how every cell in the body works. However, too much cholesterol in the blood can increase your relative's risk of heart problems. Cholesterol is carried around the body by proteins. The combinations of cholesterol and proteins are called lipoproteins. There are two main types of lipoproteins: LDL (low-density lipoprotein), which is the harmful type of cholesterol and HDL (high-density lipoprotein), which is a protective type of cholesterol. Having too much harmful LDL cholesterol in the blood can increase the risk of cardiovascular disease. The risk is particularly high if your relative has a high level of LDL cholesterol and a low level of HDL cholesterol.

Triglycerides are another type of fatty substance in the blood. They are found in foods such as dairy products, meat and cooking oils. They can also be produced in the body, either by the body's fat stores, or in the liver. People who are very overweight, eat a lot of fatty and sugary foods, or drink too much alcohol are more likely to have a high triglyceride level and have a greater risk of developing cardiovascular disease than those with lower levels.

A common cause of high blood cholesterol levels is eating too much saturated fat. However, some people have high blood cholesterol even though they eat a healthy diet. For example, they may have inherited a condition called familial hyperlipidemia (FH). The cholesterol which is found in some foods, such as eggs, liver, kidneys and some types of seafood, e.g. prawns, does not usually make a great contribution to the level of cholesterol in your blood. It is much more important that you eat foods that are low in saturated fat, such as fruit, vegetables, wholegrains, poultry, fish and nuts.

My father suffered from high cholesterol due to familial hyperlipidemia. When on holiday in Florida, he took a cholesterol test in the pharmacy – it was a novelty at the time as such a test was not yet available over the counter in the UK – and the level was so high that the pharmacist told him to lie down in the store while they called an ambulance. My father knew the level was normal. He did not lie down and he refused to go to hospital, heading back to the beach instead.

To help reduce your relative's cholesterol level, they need to cut down on saturated fats and instead, use unsaturated fats, such as olive, rapeseed, or sunflower oils and spreads. They should also reduce the total amount of fat they eat. Oily fish provides the richest source of a particular type of polyunsaturated fat known as Omega-3. Omega-3 from oily fish can help to lower blood triglyceride levels and prevent the blood from clotting and regulate the heart rhythm. Foods that are high in soluble fibre, such as oats, beans, pulses, lentils, nuts, fruit and vegetables, can help lower cholesterol. Regular physical activity can help increase HDL cholesterol (the 'protective' type of cholesterol). There is evidence to show that substances called plant sterols and stanols may help reduce cholesterol levels when 2g per day is regularly consumed. They can be found in margarines, spreads, soft cheeses and yogurts.

For most people, there is currently no limit on the number of eggs that they can eat in a week. However, because the recommendation has changed over the years, it is often a common source of confusion. In the past, a restriction on eggs was recommended, because it was thought that foods high in cholesterol (including liver, kidneys and shellfish, as well as eggs) could have an impact on cholesterol levels in the body. However, as research in this area has developed, so has our understanding of how foods that contain cholesterol affect our heart health. For most people, the amount of saturated fat they eat has much more of an impact on their cholesterol than eating foods which contain cholesterol, like eggs and shellfish. So, unless your relative has been advised otherwise by their doctor or dietician, if they like eggs, they can be included as part of a balanced and varied diet.

Whether they need to take cholesterol-lowering drugs or not depends not just on their total cholesterol HDL and LDL levels, but also on their overall risk of cardiovascular disease. Cholesterol-lowering medicines, such as statins, are prescribed for people who are at greatest overall risk of suffering from cardiovascular disease.

Angina

Angina is a pain or discomfort felt in the chest and usually caused by coronary heart disease. However, in some cases, the pain may affect some people only in the arm, neck, stomach or jaw. Angina often feels like a heaviness or tightness in the chest, but this may spread to the arms, neck, jaw, back, or stomach as well. Some people describe a feeling of severe tightness, while others say it is more of a dull ache. Symptoms of experiencing shortness of breath have been reported too. Angina is often brought on by physical activity, an emotional upset, cold weather, or after a meal. Symptoms usually subside after a few minutes. Unfortunately, you cannot reverse coronary heart disease, but your relative can help prevent angina and the condition from getting worse by keeping their heart healthy.

It is important to stop smoking, control high blood pressure, reduce your relative's cholesterol level, be physically active, achieve and maintain a healthy weight, control blood glucose if your relative has diabetes, eat a healthy, balanced diet and only drink moderate amounts of alcohol. Their doctor may be able to diagnose whether they have angina from the symptoms that they describe. Alternatively, the GP may want to carry out a health check, or send them for some tests. There is medication available that can help control symptoms, whereas some people require angioplasty, or heart bypass surgery to clear the arteries. Many people with angina have a good quality of life and continue with their normal daily activities. Your relative's doctor or nurse will be able to advise them on daily activities and any lifestyle changes they may need to make.

If your relative experiences chest pains, call 999 immediately.

Heart attack

Most heart attacks are caused by coronary heart disease, which is when coronary arteries narrow due to a gradual build-up of fatty material (atheroma) within the walls. If the atheroma becomes unstable, a piece may break off and lead to a blood clot forming. This clot can block the coronary artery, starving the heart of blood and oxygen and causing damage to the heart muscle. This is a heart attack. It is also called acute coronary syndrome, myocardial infarction, or coronary thrombosis. A heart attack is life-threatening. If you think your relative, or anyone else, is having a heart attack, you should phone 999 for an ambulance immediately.

Top tip: You are more likely to survive a heart attack if you phone 999 straight away and receive fast treatment. Don't hesitate.

Cardiac arrest is totally different from a heart attack. A cardiac arrest happens when the heart stops pumping blood around the body. As a result, your relative will be unconscious and will not be breathing normally. Immediate cardiopulmonary resuscitation (CPR) and defibrillation is needed to have any chance of survival. One of the causes of cardiac arrest is a heart attack. Other causes include electrocution, or choking.

Top tip: If you witness a cardiac arrest, you can increase the person's chances of survival by phoning 999 and giving immediate CPR. As a carer, it is worth considering taking a first aid course, which covers CPR and trains you in how to act in emergency medical situations. St John Ambulance, the British Red Cross and other organisations all run first aid training courses.

The symptoms of a heart attack vary from one person to another. They can range from a severe pain in the centre of the chest to having mild chest discomfort that makes your relative feel generally unwell. The pain or discomfort may feel like bad indigestion. This may spread to the arms, neck, jaw, back or stomach and can also cause chest pain. Your relative can feel light-headed or dizzy and short of breath. They may also feel nauseous or vomit. Phone 999 immediately if you think someone is having a heart attack. This means that you will get potentially life-saving treatment as soon as possible. Do not phone the GP if you think someone is having a heart attack, you must dial 999 for an ambulance.

Top tip: If your relative is not allergic to aspirin and has some next to them, or if there is someone with them who can fetch some for them easily, they can chew an aspirin to try to prevent further damage to the heart muscle and increase their chances of survival. The British Heart Foundation advises that if your relative does not have aspirin to hand, they should not get up and wander around the house looking for one as this may put unnecessary strain on the heart. They should call 999 and wait for assistance from an ambulance crew.

When the ambulance staff arrives, they will do an electrocardiogram (ECG). This should not delay transfer to the most suitable hospital. The crew will administer aspirin if it has not already been given, assess your relative's symptoms and medical history, give pain relief if needed and oxygen if oxygen levels are too low. They will also examine your relative and monitor their heart rate and blood pressure. They may perform primary percutaneous coronary intervention (PPCI), which is emergency coronary angioplasty. This involves reopening the blocked coronary artery and placing one or more stents in it. It restores blood supply to the part of the heart that is starved of blood, which helps to save as much muscle as possible. A medicine is injected into the vein to dissolve the blood clot and restore the blood supply to the heart. If PPCI is not possible in the home, it will be given in the ambulance. In some types of heart attacks, people do not receive either of these two treatments, because they will not benefit from them.

Living a healthy lifestyle can help prevent your relative from having a heart attack. They should ask their doctor or nurse for a heart health check to assess their risk of having a heart attack in the next 10 years. If they have already had a heart attack, they can dramatically reduce the risk of having another one and of future heart problems by keeping their heart healthy and taking their medicines. A heart attack can be a frightening experience and it can take time to come to terms with what has happened. It is natural to be worried about recovery and the future. Many people make a full recovery and within a few months are able to return to their normal activities. Some may find that they are not able to do as much as they previously did, but attending a cardiac rehabilitation course will increase the chances of getting back to normal as quickly as possible. Ask your relative's GP or consult www.cardiac-rehabilitation.net/cardiac-rehab.htm.

Heart failure

Having heart failure means that, for some reason, the heart is not pumping blood around the body as well as it used to. The most common reason is that the heart muscle has been damaged – for example, after a heart attack. It can be very frightening to hear that your relative has heart failure. For many people, heart failure can be a debilitating condition, where normal everyday tasks, such as having a shower or bath, doing the shopping, or simply playing with the children, takes enormous energy and leaves them breathless and exhausted. There are many reasons why your relative might be diagnosed with heart failure. It can be sudden, or it may happen slowly over months, even years. Some causes of heart failure are a heart attack, high blood pressure, problems with heart valves, cardiomyopathies (diseases of the heart muscle), drinking too much alcohol and congenital conditions (those that people are born with).

Not everyone experiences the same symptoms and everyone copes in different ways. Your relative might feel out of breath when they are physically active, or in some cases, even when they are at rest. They may also have swollen feet and ankles and feel very tired. Everyone is different, so it is important to speak to their GP about what is best for them. The reason for their condition will make a difference as to how their symptoms are controlled. You may need to have tests, which include blood tests, an electrocardiogram (ECG) and an echocardiogram.

While there is no cure for heart failure at the moment, the treatment to control symptoms has improved dramatically. With treatment and the right medicines, many people live full and active lives. Your relative's doctor will prescribe drugs that will help control their blood pressure and help the pumping action of their heart. They will also give advice about making changes to their lifestyle, such as cutting down on salt, staying active and stopping smoking, which will help them to do all the things that they enjoy, improve their condition and try to live a normal life.

Heart valve disease

The heart is a muscle, which pumps blood to the lungs and around the rest of the body. There are four chambers to the heart, which are separated by valves to make sure that the blood flows in one direction through the heart. The two large blood vessels that leave the heart also have valves which ensure that the blood does not go back into the heart once it has been pumped out.

The main causes of heart valve disease are being born with an abnormal valve or valves (congenital heart disease), having had rheumatic fever, cardiomyopathy (a disease of the heart muscle), damage to the heart muscle from a heart attack, or a previous infection with endocarditis (an infection of the inner lining of the heart chambers and heart valves). A diseased or damaged valve can affect the flow of blood in two ways. If the valve does not open fully, it will obstruct the flow of blood. This is called valve stenosis, or narrowing. If the valve does not close properly, it will allow blood to leak backwards. This is called valve incompetence, regurgitation, or a leaky valve. Both will put extra strain on the heart and if your relative has stenosis, the valve can restrict the flow of blood, making their heart pump harder to force the blood past the narrowing. If your relative has valve incompetence, a leaking valve may mean that their heart has to do extra work to pump the required volume of blood through the heart.

Your relative may not experience any symptoms, but if they do, some of the common symptoms are being out of breath, swelling of the ankles and feet and being unusually tired. Their doctor may hear a murmur (an unusual sound) when they listen to their heart. A murmur does not always mean that there is a problem with the heart as people with normal hearts may also have murmurs. The GP may suggest that your relative has further tests to see how well the heart is working. The most common test is an echocardiogram, which uses sound waves to look at the structure of the heart. It is similar to an ultrasound scan used to look at babies before they are born. Your relative may not need any treatment at all, but their doctor may ask them to come back in a year's time, or if symptoms get worse. Most valve problems, however, can be treated using medicines or by surgery. The treatment will depend on the cause of the problem and the effect that it is having on the heart.

You can find more information on heart-related illness and prevention at British Heart Foundation (www.bhf.org.uk).

Hip and knee replacements

Hips

A worn hip means that the bones rub together and cause considerable pain. A replacement involves removing this bone and replacing it with new pieces, made from either metal, plastic or ceramic. Hip replacements last between 10 and 20 years and should reduce or eliminate pain and increase mobility. A replacement also reduces dependency on painkillers and anti-inflammatory drugs.

Replacement hips can be either cemented, known as 'fixed', or un-cemented. Fixed hips tend to be given to older people, who hopefully will not need a second replacement in their lifetime. A second hip replacement is known as a 'revision'. In un-cemented hips, metal surfaces can be treated with a substance and roughened to encourage the bone growth into the artificial joint and fix it in place. Metal and ceramic parts tend to be more hard-wearing and more common now as metal-on-metal implants tend to wear out faster and need future hip revisions. Hip revisions can be more complicated than the original hip replacements, as they require removal of the first hip replacement and some bone will be lost. It can take longer to recover from revisions. If you are under 65, hip resurfacing might be an option, which is where damaged bone is removed and the ball and socket are covered with metal caps. First hip operations are often now performed as keyhole surgery, but this is not possible for revisions.

Prior to having a hip operation, there are a few things to bear in mind. Smoking increases the risk of chest and wound infection and can slow recovery. Losing weight reduces the pressure on your relative's hip and may help to speed up recovery. When visiting the specialist, it can be a good idea to make a list before you go with your relative, so that you do not forget to ask anything while you are in the appointment.

A hip replacement operation usually takes about an hour and a half to perform and can be done using an epidural as a spinal block, which means you are awake during the procedure, but can feel nothing below the waist. In this instance, your relative does not need to recover from a general anaesthetic. If they do have general anaesthetic, they will not be allowed to eat or drink for about six hours beforehand. The surgeon and anaesthetist will advise on the right procedure for them. Hip revision surgery can take longer. To avoid blood clots forming in the veins in the legs after surgery and causing deep vein thrombosis (DVT), your relative will probably be asked to wear compression stockings, which are normally supplied by the hospital. They might also be given drugs to prevent DVT. When they wake up, they may find a pillow between their legs to hold the hip joint still and prevent dislocation. They will be given painkillers.

Your relative will usually get physiotherapy treatment very soon after their operation and regularly afterwards for a while. They will be given exercises to restore movement and will be expected to stand within 24 hours of the operation and walk not long after that. It is very important to do the exercises the physiotherapist prescribes. Your relative is usually in hospital for three to five days and will be discharged when they can walk easily with crutches or a stick (see pages 92–94 for details on hospital discharge). They may have stitches which need to be removed, or they might have dissolvable stitches, which do not need removing. Your relative should be prescribed painkillers to take at home when they leave hospital and they will need to continue with their physiotherapy exercises. It is important not to cross the legs or twist the hip as it may strain the scar or even dislocate the new hip. They will need help at home getting in and out of bed and chairs and going to the toilet. Ideally someone should stay with your relative on their return until they are well enough to cope on their own, but hospitals are not always able to arrange this, so it is usually a family member.

Top tip: Using a heightened toilet seat extension can often be very helpful, so your relative does not have to squat as deeply as usual while recovering at home after a hip replacement. The hospital should provide this if you ask.

Your relative will not be able to drive for a while and how quickly they can return to driving will depend on which leg has been operated on and if they have a manual or an automatic car. Once recovered, they may need to avoid sports, which have a risk of being hit hard or even falling.

There may be complications with hip surgery. Infection can occur, but your relative will be given antibiotics after surgery to prevent this. Post-surgery, one leg may be slightly longer or shorter than the other, but this can be corrected with orthotics in their shoes. Dislocation and fractures can occur, but are rare.

My husband had a hip replacement. Originally, his leg had been an inch shorter than the other due to an accident in childhood. After the operation, when the nurses stood him up, he banged his leg hard on the floor because the surgeon had now made it an inch longer. It took him a while to get used to it and the change in leg length has created additional back problems for him.

The NHS has further information at www.nhs.uk/conditions/hip-replacement.

Knees

If your relative's quality of life is severely restricted due to knee pain and immobility, they may wish to consider a knee replacement. The operation is rarely an emergency and is generally their choice. Typical symptoms which may mean they need knee replacement surgery include pain, which gradually gets worse over time, and having sudden acute attacks of pain. The pain is normally worse when weight-bearing and doing any normal activity. Swelling can be severe and prevent your relative from bending their knee. They should see their doctor to rule out any infection, especially if they have a fever. Knees can be stiff in the morning in particular, but may improve slightly during the day. This is particularly prevalent in people with rheumatoid arthritis. Being overweight makes knee pain worse. Carrying too much weight puts extra stress on the joints and can make symptoms of arthritis considerably worse.

There are two types of knee replacement: total and partial. Total knee replacement requires an incision over the knee and usually entails a hospital stay of a few days to a week. Recovery can take from one to three months, but the good news is that most patients are free of their arthritic symptoms once they have recovered. Partial knee replacement is less invasive, but is only suitable for about 10 per cent of all patients. This is suitable for someone who only has arthritis in one of the three knee compartments. Your relative's GP will refer them to an orthopaedic surgeon, who will examine them, as well as looking at their medical history and taking X-rays, which will clearly show any arthritis. X-rays taken standing up are preferable as they show what happens to the knee when it is weight-bearing. More than 90 per cent of people who have total knee replacements have no pain after recovery, or substantially less pain. Replacements also relieve stiffness and enable them to live normal active lives.

Physiotherapy usually begins on the day of surgery, or on the day afterwards. Patients are encouraged to walk and to weight-bear as much as they can. They will also be given exercises to do regularly. Immediately after getting home, they may need help getting around, getting out of bed, or going to the toilet. Having grab rails in the bathroom and by the bed can be very helpful. Physiotherapy will normally continue after discharge from hospital and your relative can also do exercises at home. The aim is to get to at least a 90-degree knee bend within two weeks of surgery. After about a month, most people can move about well and will be back to normal after three months.

After recovery, it is a good idea to walk, swim and do other exercises to keep fit, keep weight off and keep the knees supple. Running is usually not recommended with a total knee replacement.

My sister had both knees replaced at the same time and her recovery was long and difficult. She ended up being admitted back into hospital for quite a while. My mother had her knees replaced individually, one year apart, and her recovery was much faster, despite being 30 years older than my sister.

The NHS has further information at www.nhs.uk/conditions/knee-replacement.

Incontinence

Older people suffering with incontinence can often be too embarrassed to come forward and seek help for it. They do not find it an easy subject to discuss with relatives or medical staff. However, it is really important that if someone does have problems getting to the toilet on time that they should ask for help. It is not something they should have to cope with alone, or that cannot be resolved and it is important to recognise that these problems are common and nothing to be ashamed of.

When seeing healthcare staff about a bladder or bowel problem, your relative should be seen and examined by a nurse or doctor, who is trained to do an assessment and then they might be referred to a specialist, who is able to answer questions relating to incontinence problems, can provide a diagnosis and discuss all available treatments. Staff should always treat the patient with sensitivity. This can be a distressing time and your relative should be made to feel as comfortable as possible at all times. They may wish to take a chaperone, although some people prefer to go alone. Make sure that different treatment options are explained, as well as what they can do to help themselves. There are also patient groups they can join.

When visiting healthcare staff about bladder or bowel problems, the staff should ask about what the symptoms are and about other medical conditions which may be contributing to the bowel or bladder problem. Medication can be a cause. Your relative will possibly have tests for infection and may be asked to record the frequency of toilet visits. There may also be an internal examination to check for prolapse in women and prostate issues in men. Again, your relative may wish to take a chaperone, although some people prefer to go alone.

It may be helpful to reduce caffeine intake and to drink more fluids to aid constipation. There are incontinence pads on sale in all leading supermarkets and chemists, as well as on numerous websites. Many of these products come as pull-up pants, so they can be worn as underwear. Barrier cream, such as Sudocrem, is helpful to protect and soothe the skin. Try to encourage your relative to go to the bathroom regularly to avoid accidents and to plan ahead for trips and visits outside the home and take products with them. They can keep a bag packed with pads, cream, wipes, etc. ready to go. Stopping smoking is important, as this can make the bladder over-active. Pelvic floor muscle exercises are often very effective in treating urinary incontinence. These exercises, also known as Kegel exercises, are aimed at strengthening the bladder's sphincter and therefore allowing it to seal off the bladder better. Sphincter muscles are part of a group called the pelvic floor muscles. Strengthening the pelvic floor reflects positively on the strength of the sphincter and greatly improves stress incontinence.

The NHS offers further information at www.nhs.uk/conditions/urinary-incontinence.

Managing medication

Medication often plays an important role in older people's health and ensuring that the people you care for take it at the right time, in the right way and with the right frequency and dosage, is essential. Medication should be taken as directed by a doctor or pharmacist, or according to the instructions on the packet. This ensures your relative achieves the full benefit of the medication and lessens any possible side effects. Try to make sure that thay take their medication at the same time every day.

Some medicines need to be taken at specific times, such as before, with, or after food. The management of certain medical conditions, such as Parkinson's disease, can only be controlled with very precise, set dosage timings, so it may help to set reminders on a calendar, phone, or in a special app on your or their smartphone or tablet. Medication that is out of date should never be taken. In the event a dose is missed, do not take another or give a double dose to make up for the missed dose. Check the patient information leaflet in the medication packaging, which your relative should always keep until the medication is finished as there is usually a section which relates to missed doses, though it is recommended that you speak to a pharmacist to get the best advice. It is a good idea to keep the phone number of the pharmacy and doctor's surgery in your phone or diary (see page 25 for a list of useful numbers to keep). When a new medication is prescribed, always ask your doctor for the appropriate course of action if a dose is missed. If doses are missed regularly, start to keep a medication diary of what your relative has taken and not taken (and why, if known) and discuss it with their GP as soon as possible.

It is very important to inform the doctor of all other medication that your relative might be taking in order to ascertain how all the drugs might interact together and to discuss possible side effects and things to watch out for. It is also a good idea to meet with the GP regularly to ensure all medication is still needed.

The doctor only ever prescribes a limited course of medication, so it is sensible to make a note in your relative's or your diary, or set a reminder on your phone, to order a repeat prescription a week before it is due to run out. Check with the GP's surgery to find out how many days the practice needs to process repeat prescription requests. Most GPs now offer a dedicated telephone line for repeat prescription ordering, or an online web service and some pharmacies offer a convenient repeat prescription service, where you let them know what medicines your relative needs and they will arrange the repeat prescription with the GP practice for you and in some cases, deliver the medication to your relative directly.

Medication can deteriorate and not work as intended if exposed to heat, light or moisture. It is best not to keep medicines in a damp or steamy place, such as a kitchen or bathroom, or on windowsills. Medication is best stored in a cool, dark place. However, always check the label for special storage instructions, such as 'store in the fridge' or 'away from sunlight'. Try to keep all medication together in one place for ease of access unless there are specific instructions for storage. Medicines stored in the fridge are best placed in a separate container (e.g. a plastic box or resealable bag) and kept away from food and other consumables. If the person you care for does not live alone, make sure that medication for each person in the home is stored separately, so that they do not get mixed up. Always keep medication out of the reach of children. It is important to store medicines in their original containers and packaging, along with their instructions for use. Do not decant medication into other containers as they may get mixed up and taken accidentally.

Many people need help with medication from carers due to poor eyesight, or if they are registered blind. If the person you care for is unable to read the directions on their medication packaging, ask the pharmacist to provide them in large print and to talk through the instructions as well. If the person you care for is registered blind, it is important that new supplies of medication are checked for any brand changes, which may be in different sized outer packaging, or have different shaped tablets. Speak to the pharmacist, who may be able to ensure generic brands are always provided, so that the tablet shape remains familiar and consistent and this will help to prevent medication errors. There are some specialised apps available, which will connect blind people with sighted volunteers who can help with medication labelling – among other things – via video link. Labels can be provided in Braille for blind or partially sighted patients.

If you care for someone with swallowing difficulties, or someone who has to chew tablets before swallowing, speak to the pharmacist about suitable soluble and liquid alternatives. You can also use a pill crusher to halve and/or crush pills and tablets to make them easier to take. A dry mouth makes it harder to swallow, so it's a good idea to moisten the mouth with water first. Place the tablet in the centre of the tongue and lengthways along the tongue if the pill is oval-shaped. Immediately, take a sip of water and wash the pill directly into the throat, throwing the head back.

Top tip: Try getting your relative to use a straw to drink the water as the suction may help them to swallow tablets.

There are options available for people who have dexterity difficulties when taking medication. A blister pack pen device is easy to hold and helps your relative to get into a medication blister pack more easily. A Haleraid, or other inhaler aids, are available for those who are arthritic, or have difficulty depressing an inhaler. If an eye drop bottle is too small to squeeze a drop from, there are dispensers designed for arthritic hands. A winged cap is a simple device that is placed onto the top of a medication bottle to help open it. If your relative has memory problems, having a medication record with pictures of the medication and an explanation of all the medicines to be taken, including when they should be taken, how many and what they are for, can help as a useful prompt. These can be on paper, or in electronic form. People who have difficulty remembering if they have taken tablets may benefit from a medication diary or tick chart. If ticked when tablets are taken, these charts can be a good way of reminding them that tablets have been taken, but they are obviously inappropriate if a patient is unaware of the day and time. Managing medication for someone who needs to take a variety of pills every day is a critical task as it is important to ensure the correct dosage and timing. Modern pill dispensers can be pre-loaded with a day's, or a week's worth of medication, and will automatically dispense the right medication at the right time by sending out an alert, or sounding an alarm, to show that the medication is ready to take. You can also buy standard pill boxes to pre-allocate medication by days of the week.

For people with more pronounced memory issues, electronic medicines dispensers audibly and visibly remind them to take their medicines. These are locked within the device, so they can only take medicines at the times at which the alarm has been set.

Pharmacists are medicine experts and will be happy to help you with any medication queries you may have. In England & Wales, pharmacists provide a free medicines use review (MUR) service. This may benefit you and the people you care for by providing a review of all medicines to see if there are any overlaps or interactions, and they can provide extra information on what medicines are for and their side effects. Your local pharmacy can often provide a medication delivery service or collection of unwanted medicines and provide advice on compliance aids to assist with taking medicines. It will make it easier for your pharmacist to talk to you about the medicines of the person you care for if they know you are a carer and have written consent from the person for whom you care. You can also call NHS direct on 111.

Important: Do not throw away unwanted or expired medication with your normal rubbish, or wash it down the sink or toilet. Take any medicines that the person you care for no longer needs, or are out of date, back to your local pharmacy. Do not keep them 'just in case'. After a medication is changed or discontinued, the remaining supplies should be returned to your pharmacy to be disposed of safely.

In the event a person dies, keep their medication for at least seven days in case the Coroner's Office, Procurator Fiscal or Courts ask for them. Always dispose of medication which has reached its expiry date. Remember, some medication expires sooner once it has been opened, such as eye drops. Write the date your relative opened them on the packaging, so you can keep track of when they are due to expire.

Pain management

It is thought that much pain in the older population often goes under-reported due to stoicism. Older people tend to put up with severe discomfort and pain because they do not wish to be a nuisance. Unfortunately, not addressing pain can have negative long-term consequences, including reduced mobility and depression, and so managing pain in older people is critical.

The first step is to visit the GP to get a proper diagnosis and medical opinion. If your relative is otherwise healthy, then painkillers will normally be prescribed. Of course, some older people genuinely dislike taking painkillers and if this is the case, there are other approaches to managing and reducing pain. There are around 300 pain clinics in the UK, mostly located in hospitals staffed by multi-disciplinary teams, including occupational therapists, psychologists, doctors, and physiotherapists, who work together to help people with pain. The aim is to help them manage chronic pain and maintain a good quality of life.

Remaining physically active as you age is vital to staying healthy and maintaining independence. Regular exercise is known to improve general health, help maintain a healthy weight and to reduce the risk of falls, heart disease and stroke. It also helps to reduce and manage pain. Even if your relative has never been particularly sporty or interested in exercising, it is not too late to start. It is important for older people to keep moving and avoid spending too many hours sitting down. There are many ways to get physical exercise, such as walking, gardening, golf, bowls, tennis, swimming, dancing, Tai Chi and yoga (see pages 118–123 for ideas). Older people are recommended to do around two to three hours of moderate-intensity aerobic activity every week, with a target of achieving 30 minutes on at least five days a week. At least two days a week, activities should focus on strengthening muscles. One of the benefits of regular exercise is that it helps people to relax and proper relaxation can help to reduce stress caused by chronic pain. There are many relaxation techniques that older people can try, from breathing exercises to meditation. The important thing here is that regular practice should help to reduce pain. Their GP should be able to offer advice and there may be local classes they can attend. Exercise also helps with depression as it releases endorphins, which improve your mood.

Physiotherapy can help maintain physical function and enhance psychological and social wellbeing, so reducing pain. Importantly, physiotherapy includes specific exercises designed to improve or increase coordination, flexibility, endurance, balance, strength and general range of motion. This all helps to improve circulation, reduce pain and the risk of falls. Physiotherapy is available through the NHS (via a GP referral), through the voluntary sector, and privately (see also pages 123–124). Acupuncture too can be very effective in managing pain in older people. It uses ultra-fine sterile needles inserted into specific parts of the body to rebalance energy, promote self-healing, and reduce pain.

Acupuncture is sometimes available on the NHS, so it is worth checking with your relative's GP (see pages 129–130).

Sometimes, simply shifting one's focus onto something else can help take one's mind off moderate pain. Depending on what your relative is interested in, you can try suggesting activities, such as watching TV, going to the cinema, visiting a friend, listening to music, doing a crossword, or spending time enjoying a favourite hobby, such as singing, knitting or photography. Going out for the day can also provide stimulation and company that helps to distract from dwelling too much on aches and pains.

You can get more information from The British Pain Society at www.britishpainsociety.org/people-with-pain.

Parkinson's disease

Parkinson's is a progressive neurological condition. One person in every 500 has Parkinson's. Most people who get Parkinson's are aged 50 or over, but younger people can get it too. One in 20 is under the age of 40. People with Parkinson's do not have enough of a chemical called dopamine, because some nerve cells in their brain have died. Without dopamine, people can find that their movements become slower, so it takes longer to do things. The loss of nerve cells in the brain cause the symptoms of Parkinson's to appear. There is currently no cure for Parkinson's and it is not yet known why people get the condition. Parkinson's does not directly cause people to die, but symptoms do become worse over time.

The main symptoms of Parkinson's are tremor, rigidity and slowness of movement. People with Parkinson's can find that other issues, such as tiredness, pain, depression and constipation, have an impact on their day-to-day lives. Bladder problems may occur in Parkinson's, as it affects the nerves that control emptying the bladder. This can lead to an overactive bladder and the need to pass urine more often and quickly. Some people with Parkinson's may get constipation, which can make them feel unwell, lethargic and even nauseous, but it rarely leads to serious complications. Increasing the amount of water they drink and how much fibre they eat, following a balanced diet and taking regular exercise will stimulate the bowel to help prevent constipation. Some people with Parkinson's may find they have problems when eating and saliva can build up in the mouth, which sometimes overflows. Practising keeping lips together, learning tips on tongue control and other similar exercises may help with any difficulties in swallowing and may also help to control drooling. In some cases, changing posture and sitting more upright can improve matters. You can find out more at www.parkinsons.org.uk.

Loss of balance and falling can be common in Parkinson's. Falls are caused by many factors, such as the changes in posture that may happen as Parkinson's progresses. Some people with Parkinson's will experience freezing, stopping suddenly while walking and feeling as if their feet are glued to the ground. They may then be unable to move forward again for several seconds or even minutes. It is not known exactly what causes freezing, but it may happen when movements are interrupted, or when the movement is just starting. Freezing does not just affect walking. It can also occur during repetitive movements, like writing or brushing teeth. There may be problems with different kinds of communication, including speech, facial expressions and writing. Many people with Parkinson's have some speech problems when they first develop the condition. These may make everyday activities, such as talking to friends or using the phone, difficult. The speech problems that some people with Parkinson's have may be helped by speech and language therapy.

Eye problems, such as blurred or double vision, dry eyes or excessive watering, can be common for people with Parkinson's. Some of these issues will be due to Parkinson's, or the treatment they are receiving. If they experience any eye problems, they should see the GP, specialist or Parkinson's nurse. Parkinson's can also cause the sweat glands to overreact. This can lead to too much or too little sweat, or to extremely dry skin. Changes in medication can often reduce excess sweating and ensure that the body produces enough perspiration. Dry skin and scalp problems can be irritating, but are often manageable with creams and medicated shampoos. Having a balanced diet is an important part of looking after health. With Parkinson's, the patient may need to take a little extra care, as some symptoms and side effects of treatment can limit or upset the appetite. Being underweight or overweight can have an impact on health generally.

There are many different types of pain related to this disease – for example, headaches or muscular and joint pain. Not everyone with Parkinson's experiences the same symptoms. For some people, pain can be the main symptom of their condition, although not everyone will experience this problem. It is important that both people with Parkinson's and their carers are aware of the problems pain may cause. To be able to treat pain in Parkinson's, the GP, specialist or Parkinson's nurse needs to find out what is causing the pain. In the early stages of Parkinson's, many people complain of certain difficulties in thinking and memory that can interfere with day-to-day life. This can be experienced as a slowing down of thinking, much in the same way as they might experience slowing down of movement. While some people do complain of forgetfulness, memory problems are not usually a significant complaint in the early stages of Parkinson's. It is more likely that other factors, such as stress, depression and poor general health, will have an impact on the ability to think, recall and process information efficiently. A diagnosis of Parkinson's dementia is given if the symptoms of dementia appear after those of Parkinson's. Symptoms of dementia can include slowness of thinking, poor recall, impaired concentration and talking less. Memory problems, such as forgetfulness and repetitive questioning, can also be experienced. However, some people can have dementia with hardly any memory problems. In general, people with Parkinson's dementia find they have problems with judgement and problem solving. This means it is difficult for them to make complex decisions. Activities of daily living, such as dressing, hygiene, cooking and cleaning, may also become increasingly difficult. Extra help from carers may be necessary.

Some people with Parkinson's have anxiety related to the on/off state of their motor symptoms. When off and less able to move well, they may develop significant anxiety symptoms and at times may even have panic attacks. If anxiety is related to movement problems, then talking to a doctor about altering anti-Parkinson's medication can help. For anxiety symptoms which do not respond to changes in anti-Parkinson's medication, a trial of either talk therapy, such as cognitive behavioural therapy (CBT), or medication, may be helpful. For those who experience mild anxiety every now and then, avoiding stimulants, such as caffeine, alcohol and cigarettes, can help. Some people can find relaxation tapes, yoga, massage, acupuncture and complementary therapies beneficial.

Hallucinations are rare, but some people with Parkinson's may experience complex visual hallucinations. Typically, these involve seeing small animals, insects, or other people in the room. The length of the hallucination varies and is usually visual. Auditory hallucinations are rarer for those with Parkinson's. Sometimes, when people with Parkinson's hallucinate, they experience a feeling that an animal or object is present, just next to them, but they do not actually see it. Hallucinations are caused partly by Parkinson's itself and partly by the medication that is prescribed to treat it. Dopamine and anticholinergic drugs are more likely to cause hallucinations. If your relative is experiencing hallucinations, it is important that they visit their doctor so that the cause can be identified and any appropriate treatment given. The symptoms can be controlled using a combination of drugs, therapies and, occasionally, surgery. As Parkinson's progresses, an increased amount of care and support may be required, although many people maintain a good quality of life with limited care or treatment.

Parkinson's UK has more information at www.parkinsons.org.uk.

Pneumonia

Pneumonia is usually the result of an infection, where germs multiply and cause lung infections. This is more likely to happen if your relative is already frail, or in poor health. This inflammation causes the alveoli (tiny air sacs in the lungs) to become full of fluid and as a result, the lungs struggle to work properly. In response, the brain sends white blood cells to the lungs to fight the infection, which helps kill the germs causing the infection, but also inhibits the passage of oxygen from the lungs into the bloodstream. Pneumonia is not the same as bronchitis, which is an inflammation or infection of the large airways, known as the bronchi. It is possible to get bronchitis and pneumonia at the same time, known as bronchopneumonia. Pneumonia can be caused by various bacteria, viruses or fungi. The most common bacteria are called Streptococcus Pneumonia. Pneumonia spreads via infection from person to person, as it is an airborne infection. It can develop from flu, particularly in older people, as flu lowers the immune system.

If your relative has pneumonia, they will have similar symptoms to flu or a chest infection, but symptoms often develop more quickly. These will include a high or very high temperature, shivering, sweating and coughing, which produces dark yellow or green phlegm, sometimes flecked with blood. They may also experience rapid breathing, which if too rapid, can be a sign of the severity of pneumonia, as well as disorientation and confusion and a sharp pain in the side of the chest, worse with deep breathing, which can mean that pleurisy has developed. Pleurisy is when the thin outer covering of the lung becomes infected and inflamed by pneumonia. If they are suffering any of these symptoms, seek medical help immediately.

People who are in hospital with other problems sometimes develop pneumonia while they are there. This does not mean that the hospital is unhygienic, simply that their resistance to the germs that can cause pneumonia has been weakened by their other medical problems. To avoid catching pneumonia, your relative should try to stop smoking. Smokers have an increased risk of developing pneumonia, as well as other chest infections. It is important to practice good hygiene to reduce the spread of germs, so encourage them to use a tissue and hand sanitisers when they cough or sneeze and to dispose of it immediately. They must wash their hands regularly too. It is a very good idea to get a flu jab, which is available from their GP, or from many pharmacists. The flu jab is free for anyone over the age of 65. You can also vaccinate older people against pneumonia. The pneumococcal polysaccharide vaccine (PPV) is available for people aged 65+ and anyone over the age of two, who fall into a high-risk category. It is usually only needed as a one-off vaccine.

The doctor will diagnose pneumonia based on the symptoms described above, or if necessary, using a chest X-ray. The main treatment for pneumonia is antibiotics. In addition, it is important to get plenty of rest and to drink ideally eight glasses of water per day. Painkillers will almost certainly be prescribed to alleviate headaches and other aching and pain. Some people with mild pneumonia manage at home with treatment from the GP while others need to go to hospital, where they will be given antibiotics and fluids intravenously by drip into a vein. Oxygen may also be provided. Seriously ill patients, who are struggling to breathe, may be put on a ventilator, which moves air in and out of the lungs if a person is unable to breathe normally.

If pneumonia is mild, your relative may be ill for a week or so and slowly get back to normal, followed by a steady return to normal activity. With severe pneumonia, requiring hospitalisation, it might take weeks or months for them to feel fully well again. Most people recover from pneumonia and return to good health, but between 5 and 14 per cent of people who are admitted to hospital with pneumonia sadly die, many of them older.

You can get further information from the NHS at www.nhs.uk/conditions/pneumonia.

Prostate

The prostate gland is a part of the male reproductive system. It is about the size of a walnut and sits below the bladder, surrounding the urethra, which is the tube that carries urine and semen from the bladder to the penis. Its main function is to produce seminal fluid. When many men reach the age of 40, their prostates begin to get bigger and can cause problems when urinating. This is usually a non-cancerous, treatable condition, known as benign prostatic hyperplasia (BPH). According to the NHS, prostate cancer is the most common cancer in men in the UK, with more than 40,000 new cases diagnosed every year, which is more than 110 men every day. Across the UK, around 250,000 men are currently living with prostate cancer. When cells in the prostate grow faster than normal in an uncontrolled way, this can result in a tumour. In the early stages, the tumour is hard to detect, as it cannot be seen, grows slowly, and often causes no symptoms for years.

It is important to note that the symptoms of growths in the prostate are very similar, whether they are cancerous or benign (BPH). Most prostate cancers (80 per cent) grow slowly and may not cause any symptoms or illness. Symptoms may only be noticed when the prostate is large enough to put pressure on the urethra and causes problems with urination. However, in 20 per cent of cases, the prostate cancer cells can grow more quickly and may spread to other parts of the body. Men are often very reluctant to get their prostate checked, usually out of embarrassment, but the test is usually just a blood test and it can save your life, so encourage your male relative to have it done.

Common symptoms for prostate problems (both BPH and cancer) may include increased need to urinate, often during the night, needing to rush to the toilet, difficulty in starting to urinate, straining while urinating, a weak flow of urine, or feeling the bladder has not fully emptied. Rarer symptoms may include pain when urinating and finding blood in the urine or semen. Symptoms that the cancer may have spread include bone and back pain, loss of appetite, pain in the testicles and unexplained weight loss.

If symptoms become worrying, a visit to the GP is needed. The doctor will probably do a blood test and rectal examination. The blood test is taken to check for levels of a protein called prostate specific antigen (PSA), which is made in the prostate. It is normal to find some PSA in a man's bloodstream – this is called the PSA level. The PSA level reading generally increases as men get older. If the PSA level is slightly raised, the GP will usually request a second blood test is done one to three months later to check if the PSA level is rising or staying the same. A high PSA level is usually due to non-cancerous prostate enlargement (BPH), but very high PSA levels usually indicate that cancer is present and the GP will refer the patient to a specialist for an appointment within two weeks, in line with NHS guidelines. To check the prostate for any abnormal signs, including lumps, the GP will perform a digital rectal examination (DRE), which involves putting a gloved finger in the patient's back passage, or rectum. The GP may then refer the patient to hospital for more diagnostic tests. These may include rectal ultrasound, needle biopsy and an MRI scan.

If prostate cancer is detected at an early stage, then treatment is not always immediately necessary for some men. In these cases, the patient will be carefully monitored. If treatment is recommended, it will usually include surgery to remove the prostate, followed by radiotherapy and hormone therapy. As the side effects of these treatments can include erectile dysfunction and urinary incontinence, many men often choose to delay treatment. Newer treatments such as high-intensity focused ultrasound (HIFU) and cryotherapy, which have reduced side effects, may be offered by some hospitals. If the cancer is diagnosed at a later stage, it may have already spread to other parts of the body (often the bones) and cannot be cured. Treatment in these cases focuses on prolonging life and relieving the symptoms.

Prostate cancer and its treatment may cause physical changes (including extreme tiredness, bowel and bladder problems, and erectile dysfunction) as well as emotional issues. Patients should allow time to convalesce and come to terms with their experiences.

You can find out more at Prostate Cancer UK (https://prostatecanceruk.org).

Shingles

Shingles is a nerve infection, which also affects the surrounding surface connected to the nerve. Shingles comes from the same virus as chickenpox (the herpes virus), but your relative can still get it, even if they have had chickenpox as a child, as the virus remains dormant in the central nervous system. The inactive virus may not cause problems for years, if ever. Your relative cannot get shingles if they have not had chickenpox. One third of the population develops shingles and the older you are, the more common it is. It is most common in people over the age of 50, with half of all cases occurring over the age of 60 years. Most people only get shingles once. Age, a lowered immune system, cancer and its related treatments, other medication and stress can all lead to shingles.

Shingles appear as blisters in one or more bands on one side of the body, usually around the waist, or on one side of the face. The blisters normally appear a few days after the pain and initial rash. Sometimes the blisters join together, so they resemble a large burn. New blisters can keep appearing for up to a week, but will gradually heal. There may be minor scarring. An episode could last between two to four weeks. The pain from shingles can be mild to severe and may include burning, shooting pain or itching. The pain can sometimes last for months after the blisters have healed. In addition, your relative may experience a temperature, headache, nausea, upset stomach, difficulty passing urine, joint pain, swollen glands and generally feel tired and unwell. It can also affect their sense of taste and give ear and eye problems. Most adults with the dormant virus will never experience an outbreak of shingles, unless an unknown trigger activates the virus.

It is normally easy for a doctor to diagnose shingles from looking at the skin and blood tests are not usually necessary. It is important to keep the rash dry and clean to avoid infection, to wear loose-fitting clothing, which will not irritate the skin, and to use non-adherent dressings if your relative needs to cover the rash. Adhesive dressing and antibiotic dressings will irritate the rash further. Calamine lotion can help to soothe and alleviate the itching. Antihistamines may be helpful to alleviate night-time itching. Painkillers can reduce the pain. Your doctor may prescribe antiviral medicine, such as Aciclovir, to help prevent the virus from spreading. It is thought that if someone has been vaccinated against chickenpox, they are less likely to develop shingles, although this is not always the case.

The NHS has more information at www.nhs.uk/conditions/shingles.

Skin

The skin forms a natural protective barrier that, as we age, becomes less effective. It is more prone to becoming dry and less robust when exposed to irritants, such as soaps, shower gels and biological washing powders. However, by following a few simple skin care strategies, it is possible to keep the skin healthy and to avoid many of the unpleasant symptoms that can accompany the older skin.

Healthy skin can be likened to a brick wall structure, where the skin cells are the bricks, which are held together by a complex mixture of fatty acids. When there are not enough of these fatty acids, the structure of the brick wall becomes unstable. Water is lost from the skin's surface, leading to dry skin, and irritants can penetrate through the skin more easily.

There are two key ways of ensuring that the brick wall structure is kept strong. First, avoid substances which irritate the skin. These tend to break down the natural fatty acids and lead to itching and dryness. The skin may also become sore. Detergents and soaps are two of the main culprits. Normal perfumed soaps and bubble baths will cause skin dryness and are best avoided in the older person. Soap substitutes are now commonly available in chemists; broadly speaking, these are formulated in such a way as to moisturise the skin, rather than dry it. Aqueous cream has been a commonly used soap substitute; however, this has been shown to be irritating, so other non-perfumed white creams are better options. Aqueous cream should not be used as a leave-on emollient either. Other substances which will irritate the skin include washing-up liquid, cleaning products, laundry detergents and fabric conditioners. Protective gloves should always be worn when these substances are in use.

Always apply a moisturiser to the skin. There are dozens of products on the market, so it is important to find one that suits you. Greasy ointments can be helpful for very dry skin, but most people find them too sticky for everyday use. Creams are usually the best bet as they have a good ability to moisturise and are more cosmetically acceptable. Lotions are generally more watery and therefore, while easily absorbed, are less effective. The key is to find an unperfumed product and these tend to be the pharmaceutical grade emollients. Mostly, these are only available in pharmacies. Pump dispensers are cleaner and easier to use and most products are now available in this format. It is important that moisturisers are used regularly, and always after a bath or shower.

Top tip: When applying moisturiser to the skin, do so by gently stroking rather than vigorous rubbing. The moisturiser will sink into the skin of its own accord given a few minutes.

Itchy skin is a common complaint in older people. While itchy skin may be a symptom of a more serious underlying condition, more often than not, itching is the result of dryness, so avoiding irritants and using moisturisers is enough to keep itchy skin at bay. Itchy skin is always worse when an individual is not occupied or distracted. Feeling anxious seems to heighten itching, so a vicious cycle can occur, as itching causes anxiety and this worsens the itch. Keeping busy and having something else to focus on is another strategy, along with using moisturisers, for lessening the impact of itchy skin. If these simple measures are not helping, a visit to the GP is advised so that other causes of itching can be identified.

Looking after skin in cracks and crevices is particularly important. Between toes and under skin folds are vulnerable to fungal infections – the moist, warm, dark environment makes them ideal places for fungi to take hold. Careful cleansing and drying of these areas is vital. While a fungal infection is more of a nuisance than anything else, the fact that they cause breaks in the skin mean that other, more dangerous infections can take hold.

Top tip: Drying hard-to-reach areas can be difficult, so using a cool hair dryer may be helpful, or using gauze rather than a fat towel can ensure that small gaps, especially between toes, are easier to get to.

Bedsores

Bedsores result over time from pressure on skin in contact with another surface, such as a bed or wheelchair. They are very painful, difficult to treat and often lead to life-threatening infection in older people. The human body should be constantly moving, even while we are asleep. That is why we fidget in our chairs and toss and turn in bed. When we stop moving, circulation slows down. The tissue is then deprived of oxygen and nutrients and the skin can die in less than a day, or over several weeks. Older people are at much greater risk from bedsores. Skin is thinner and more vulnerable, and therefore tears more easily. Even moving an older person from the bed into a chair can cause a bedsore. Bedsores usually occur in the areas without much muscle or fat, especially on protruding bones, such as the bottom of the spine (coccyx), shoulder blades, hips, heels and elbows. They can also occur in people with arthritis, or who have limited movement. Diabetics and paraplegics also suffer. Bedsores initially begin with an itchy or sore patch of skin, which can feel warm and might feel spongy, or possibly hard. If caught at this stage, and the pressure on the area is relieved, the bedsore will normally not develop. However, if it is not caught early on, a bedsore will become blistered and sore. If it gets worse, it will eat through all the layers of skin to make a very deep wound, which means the tissue has been destroyed. At the worst stage, bedsores can destroy bone, tendons, muscles and joints and can be fatal.

To avoid bedsores, move your relative's body at least every two hours in bed, or every 30 minutes in a wheelchair. Try special beds, pillows and mattresses (foam, air, gel or water are all good options), which can help. However, this repositioning can cause its own problems. Support underneath the legs with a foam pad or pillow from the middle of the calf to the ankle and keep knees and ankles from touching. Try not to lay older people on their hip bones. Check regularly for the first signs of sores and act quickly. The majority of people suffering from bedsores are in nursing homes. Ensure that the staff treat the bedsore as they should and are constantly checking for new ones.

Bedsores are hard to heal, but it helps to eat plenty of fruit and vegetables, or to take a vitamin C supplement to aid healing. Dark red, orange and green vegetables are especially rich in the needed nutrients and nutritional supplements of vitamin C and zinc can also be helpful. Clean open sores with saltwater when you change the dressing. This helps to remove dead, damaged or infected tissue. The right dressings can help speed the healing process and protect the wound. Keep surrounding skin dry and the wound moist. Transrelative, semi-permeable dressings retain moisture and encourage new skin to grow. Infected wounds can be treated with topical antibiotics. Surgery is a last resort option and it can be very difficult to recover afterwards.

Stroke

Each year, over 150,000 people in the UK have a stroke and it is the leading cause of severe adult disability. Stroke is a medical emergency, so the sooner you can get your relative to hospital, the better chance they will have of a good recovery. The important thing for families is to be able to recognise the signs of stroke and know what action to take.

Check for stroke with the FAST test:

- Facial drooping: A section of the face, usually only on one side, that is drooping and hard to move. This can be recognised by a crooked smile
- Arm weakness: The inability to raise one's arm fully
- Speech difficulties: An inability or difficulty to understand or produce speech
- Time: If any of the symptoms above are showing, time is of the essence; call the emergency services, or go to the hospital independently.

Sometimes the symptoms of stroke may only stay for about an hour or so, and then seem to disappear. This may be a mini stroke, otherwise known as TIA (transient ischaemic attack). TIAs may be a warning sign that a major stroke is on the way, so still ring 999. It is important that you get to a TIA clinic, where the stroke risk can be assessed and managed. Forty per cent of all strokes could be avoided by the better management of high blood pressure (see pages 189–191).

Those who have a stroke and are admitted to hospital will be admitted to a stroke ward. There will be a multidisciplinary team of people, including Stroke Association Life after Stroke staff, speech and language therapists, physiotherapists and occupational therapists, who will work with the stroke survivor to support them in their recovery. Stroke can cause a wide range of disabilities but it is worth remembering that more people than ever before are making a good recovery. In fact, more than a third of stroke survivors go on to make a full recovery.

For those who are left with a disability, the most obvious problems are the physical ones, perhaps loss of mobility in their leg or arm, but the emotional impact on the stroke survivor and also the family can be just as traumatic. The sheer suddenness of a stroke turns people's lives upside down and families are left to make sense of what has happened and to create some kind of order and normality. Stroke can also affect people's ability to speak and understand what is being said. They may find it difficult to make sense of the everyday things around them and it affects their ability to connect with others. The burden of a stroke often hits home after leaving hospital. Support from the stroke team for the stroke survivor who has returned home can last up to about a year, but it is often after this time that people suddenly find themselves on their own. It is really important that stroke survivors' needs are regularly assessed. In doing so, health and social care professionals will be in a much better position to work with the stroke survivor and carer to establish what kind of treatment, care and support is needed. If this has not happened, speak to the key worker or ask your relative's GP.

The Stroke Survivor's declaration, which can be found online at www.stroke.org.uk (created for stroke survivors by stroke survivors and carers to give guidance on how to navigate the health, social care and welfare systems and what to do if the individual's needs are not being met) sets out what level of treatment, support and care people who have had a stroke should be entitled to receive. Make sure your relative's GP is aware of their changing health needs. Carers can ask to be tagged on the records as their relative's carer, so if you need to speak to the GP, you can get a carer's appointment. This can be a really helpful way of getting things moving on those occasions when they appear to be stuck.

The vast majority of strokes happen to people over the age of 65 and, consequently, they are likely to have some existing conditions, but new ones will constantly emerge. This can be the most challenging and complex of things to manage, as health services are set up to treat a range of conditions, rather than the whole person. You may find that you end up doing much of the coordination of services, as this can be the only way to move things on. It is often the seemingly small things that cause people to become trapped in their own homes. Ensure blood pressure is regularly checked to prevent a second stroke, that sight and hearing are regularly checked (stroke can affect vision and hearing), toenails are regularly clipped and teeth are OK. If a stroke sufferer seems to become confused, it is worth getting it checked out. Ill health can diminish people's world significantly and if they are unable to get out of the house, it can lead to them feeling as though their lives are of little value and hence to depression.

You can get more information from the Stroke Association at www.stroke.org.uk.

Urinary tract infection (UTI)

Urinary tract infections (UTI) can be painful and may lead to serious health problems, such as acute or chronic kidney infection, which could permanently damage the kidneys and even lead to kidney failure. They are a leading cause of sepsis, a life-threatening infection of the bloodstream. UTIs occur when bacteria in the bladder or kidney multiplies in the urine. Older people are more vulnerable to UTIs for several reasons. They are more susceptible to all infections, due to the suppressed immune system that comes with age. With age, there is also a weakening of the muscles of the bladder, which leads to more urine being retained, so the bladder does not empty properly, and they may also suffer from incontinence. The typical symptoms include cloudy urine, bloody urine, strong-smelling urine, frequent or urgent need to urinate, pain or burning with urination, pressure in the lower pelvis, low fever and night sweats, shaking or chills. Older people with serious UTIs often do not have a fever, because their immune system does not combat infection as effectively. In fact, they often do not exhibit any of the common symptoms.

> UTIs in older people are often mistaken as the early stages of dementia or Alzheimer's because symptoms are similar. People can suffer confusion or a delirium-like state, agitation, hallucinations, poor motor skills, or dizziness and a propensity to fall.

Other conditions which make the older person more susceptible to UTIs are diabetes, use of a catheter, bowel incontinence, an enlarged prostate, immobility or surgery of any area around the bladder and kidney stones. People with incontinence are more at risk from UTIs because of the close contact of incontinence pads and underwear with their skin, which can reintroduce bacteria into the bladder. Some recommendations to help reduce this risk include changing pads and underwear frequently, encouraging front-to-back cleansing and keeping the genital area clean. If possible, set reminders using timers for those who are memory-impaired to try and use the bathroom instead of incontinence underwear. Other ways to reduce the occurrence of UTIs include drinking plenty of fluids (2–4 litres every day) – drink cranberry juice, or use cranberry tablets – but avoid these if there is a history of kidney stones. Avoid caffeine and alcohol because these irritate the bladder and also avoid douches and other feminine hygiene products as they can act as irritants.

Top tip: Encourage your relative to wear cotton rather than synthetic underwear and to change it at least once a day.

If you think your relative may have a urinary tract infection, make sure they see their doctor immediately. UTIs can make older people delirious and very ill in a very short space of time.

My mother suffers from regular UTIs, but on one occasion, it progressed very quickly and by the time I arrived at her house, there was blood everywhere. It looked like a murder scene. She was taken to A&E, delirious and in great pain, and spent a week in hospital recovering. The infection became that serious within a few hours.

More information is available at the NHS website www.nhs.uk/conditions/urinary-tract-infections-utis.

Mental health

Dementia and Alzheimer's

Dementia is a very sad illness, which robs people of many of the pleasures of life. It is extremely common and will affect one in five of us who reach the age of 80. It is less common in those under 80, but some people may start with the illness in their 60s, or even earlier. It is very important to get a diagnosis and to learn to navigate your way through the various caring agencies, including the NHS, social services and the voluntary and private sectors. Dementia is probably the most difficult problem that families face when caring for an older person. Most dementia cases are caused by Alzheimer's disease, but there are other causes, including vascular dementia, Lewy body dementia (associated with Parkinson's disease) and fronto-temporal dementia. Many patients suffer from a mixture of Alzheimer's and vascular pathology. Alzheimer's disease causes 62 per cent of dementia cases in the UK.

The main area affected by Alzheimer's disease is the grey matter covering the brain, known as the cerebral cortex. This area is responsible for processing thoughts and complex functions, like retrieving and storing memories, calculation, spelling, planning and organising. It is thought that clumps of protein, known as plaques and tangles, form inside the brain. The plaques build up in the spaces between nerve cells and tangles develop inside the brain cells. Together, they interrupt the communication mechanisms between nerve cells and disrupt the processes essential to the cells' survival. Medical treatments are available to slow the onset of dementia symptoms caused by Alzheimer's disease. Cholinesterase inhibitor medications have been shown to be beneficial. These drugs make the brain cells work a little harder, thus reducing symptoms.

Vascular dementia occurs when the brain's blood supply is slowly restricted, causing brain cells to die. Alongside more common dementia symptoms, such as slower mental agility and memory loss, it can also cause muscle weakness and paralysis on one side of the body. The symptoms are similar to the symptoms of a stroke. Vascular dementia is caused by atherosclerosis, which is the narrowing and hardening of the blood vessels in the brain, which is usually a result of fatty deposits along the vessel walls. In smaller blood vessels, these fatty deposits build up, clogging the vessels and gradually depriving the brain of blood and therefore oxygen. This is known as small vessel disease. Atherosclerosis is more common in those with type 1 diabetes, high blood pressure and those who smoke. A history of stroke or small vessel disease can also increase the chances of a person developing vascular dementia.

A person with dementia with Lewy bodies will display the usual symptoms of poor memory, confusion and weaker cognitive ability, plus they may also experience alternating periods of alertness and drowsiness, fluctuating levels of confusion, visual hallucinations and less fluid physical movement. The symptoms may look similar to Parkinson's disease as the two conditions are closely related. Lewy bodies are small, circular clumps of protein that develop inside brain cells. It is unclear why they develop, or how they damage the brain, but it is thought they have an effect on the neurotransmitters that send information from one brain cell to another. The same inhibitor medications used to treat Alzheimer's disease have also shown to be beneficial in cases of dementia with Lewy bodies. By encouraging the unaffected brain cells to work harder, the medication can improve the dementia symptoms.

Fronto-temporal dementia affects the temporal lobe and frontal lobe. It typically has a greater effect on personality and behaviour. A person may seem cold and unfeeling as they have difficulty relating to the emotions of others. They may also lose their inhibitions, resulting in erratic behaviour. Language problems may occur, including loss of speech and difficulty finding the right words. This is one of the more common causes, after Alzheimer's disease, of early onset dementia. It is estimated that, in 15–40 per cent of fronto-temporal dementia cases, the person has inherited a genetic mutation from their relative.

Pick's disease is a rare type of age-related dementia that affects the frontal lobes of the brain and causes speech problems, behavioural difficulties and eventually death. It was first described by Czech neurologist and psychiatrist Arnold Pick in 1892. In some older medical texts, Pick's disease is used interchangeably with 'fronto-temporal dementia,' but in modern medicine, Pick's disease is understood to be one of three very specific causes of fronto-temporal dementia.

Parkinson's disease is caused by progressive damage to the brain resulting in tremor, slow movements and body stiffness. A person with Parkinson's disease may be diagnosed with one of two forms of dementia – Parkinson's dementia, or dementia with Lewy bodies – depending on the timing of the onset of symptoms in relation to the physical symptoms caused by Parkinson's disease (see pages 210–214).

With dementia, the first thing you may notice in your relative is memory lapse, such as an inability to name objects or people, and perhaps the beginning of more difficulty with everyday tasks, like cooking and planning. There may be incidents, such as losing the car in the car park, or failing to get off the bus at the right stop. These issues are not always caused by dementia, however. Memory problems are sometimes associated with depression, which is easily treated, or they may be worsened, or even caused by physical problems. It is important to see your relative's GP if you are worried.

Dementia is still a diagnosis that is made from your relative's clinical history and talking to them and the people who know them best, but patients also perform tests to give some clarity. They may perform a set of blood tests, including thyroid function tests, and maybe an electrocardiogram (ECG) to check the heart, as well as some cognitive tests. These tests vary, but commonly, the Mini Mental State Examination is used – where the GP asks questions, such as what day it is and who the Prime Minister is – and other more detailed tests as well. Your relative may also be offered a CT scan, or even an MRI scan, if it is felt to be necessary.

Dementia is a frightening diagnosis for the patient and for those caring for them, so you will need to learn about the illness and about the help that is available. The Alzheimer's Society (www.alzheimer.org.uk) can be very helpful, but the GP may also refer your relative to the old age psychiatry service, which will also be able to give you helpful information.

You may find it extremely trying when someone you are caring for becomes very repetitive, or is always asking the same questions. They may have odd ideas, especially if they have lost something and feel that it has been stolen, or deliberately moved. They can become aggressive and argumentative. There is not much to be gained from arguing with people in this state and it is sometimes easier for you both to accept some of what they say and only correct them when it is really necessary. As the illness progresses, patients need increasing amounts of help, particularly with personal care, and they may become very upset and angry with those trying to help them. It is important always to remember that the person living with dementia is very sensitive to his or her environment and the way in which they are treated, so they should always be offered an explanation of what is happening and be treated with gentleness and consideration. This can sometimes try the patience of a saint and carers almost always need support. You can ask for a carer assessment from your local authority to help you, and possibly to provide respite care (see pages 13–14).

Dementia is the main reason why people have to move into residential or nursing care. Although this is often a difficult decision to take, they may find the routine of institutional care reassuring and can benefit from having a larger space to wander around. Carers often feel very guilty, as eventually they cannot manage and have to let their loved one go into care, but sometimes it simply is not possible to carry on at home. The children of the person with dementia often live far away and have to try and organise the care from a distance, which is also difficult. These problems can put great pressures on families and may impact on many family relationships, so try to talk regularly and to share the load as much as you can with siblings, even if it is just helping with admin (see pages 89–92 for tips on caring from a distance).

If your relative is diagnosed with dementia, it is essential early on to grant a Lasting Power of Attorney to trusted family members or friends, so that they can make health and financial decisions on their behalf when they are no longer able to do so. Ensure your relative chooses someone they trust to look after their money and property and to make decisions about their health and wellbeing. Once a person no longer has mental capacity, Power of Attorney cannot be granted. It is also important to be sure that your relative makes a will while they are still able (see pages 27–32).

If diagnosed with dementia, your relative should try to maintain a healthy blood flow to the vessels in the brain as much as possible, by keeping blood pressure within a normal range through a healthy diet and adequate levels of exercise. If they smoke or use alcohol to excess, this can make dementia symptoms worse. For some types of dementia, specifically Alzheimer's disease and dementia with Lewy bodies, medication can be used to delay the onset of symptoms. Medication may also be useful in treating other conditions, such as vitamin B deficiency or depression, which could be making symptoms worse. Cognitive stimulation is a psychological therapy designed to help people with dementia cope with the symptoms they experience. The therapy is often completed in a group-based environment. The activities are designed to improve memory, problem-solving skills and language ability. Evidence suggests that regular engagement with cognitive stimulation therapy helps slow the deterioration caused by dementia. It is the only psychological treatment recommended by the National Institute for Health and Care Excellence (NICE). Behavioural therapy can also be helpful in the treatment of dementia. Working from the view that all behaviour is meaningful, the carer can seek to understand what drives the behaviour presented by a person with dementia, and then, with the guidance of a healthcare professional, devise a strategy to change it. For example, someone who wanders about restlessly in the early evening may not be receiving enough exercise during the day to be able to feel restful at night. One strategy to change this behaviour may be to introduce a daily walk in the afternoon.

Significant weight loss is common in people with dementia as it often affects a person's ability to make decisions and the ability to follow simple instructions, making meal planning challenging. A simple list of tried-and-trusted meal and snack ideas, especially if presented as photos rather than just words, can help a person decide what they would like to eat. A carer may need to help prepare meals. If dementia is affecting a person's ability to speak and swallow, they must seek medical advice. An inefficient swallowing mechanism can cause food particles to enter the airways, resulting in a chest infection.

It is important not to make multiple major changes to the home at once. However, there are a few minor adaptations that can be made to enable the person to live independently at home for as long as possible. Use a bright contrasting colour to make the important features of a room more visible – for example, the toilet seat, armchair – or bed linen. Keep important phone numbers on display next to the telephone (see page 25 for a list). De-clutter the home space and reduce the amount of furniture to reduce the risk of trips and falls. Ensure all rooms are well lit. A daily newspaper delivery can help a person keep track of the day and date, combined with a calendar listing all upcoming appointments and events. Reflective surfaces can be frightening for someone with dementia if they can no longer recognise their own reflection, so you may wish to cover mirrors. Written labels or photographs posted on doors and cupboards can help them to navigate around the home.

More help is available from the Alzheimer's Society (www.alzheimers.org.uk) and Dementia UK (www.dementiauk.org).

Anxiety

Anxiety issues in older people are often under-diagnosed, as older patients tend to place more emphasis on their physical problems. It used to be thought that, as we age, we become less anxious, but we now know that anxiety is just as common in old age as it is in younger age groups. Indeed, it is likely that many older people with an anxiety or panic disorder have endured the condition since they were much younger, often coping with it alone.

Anxiety is described as a feeling of unease, which can range from mild worry to severe fear. We all experience anxiety from time to time as a natural response to life events, such as exams, job interviews, public speaking, relationship problems, bereavement, moving house, etc. Severe anxiety can be caused by particular conditions, such as phobias, generalised anxiety disorder (GAD) – which is a chronic condition – post-traumatic stress disorder (PTSD), caused by distressing events, and obsessive compulsive disorder (OCD), where obsessive worries are calmed by compulsive rituals. For many older people, fear of falling can also result in severe anxiety.

Around 1 in 10 people experience occasional panic attacks, which are usually triggered by a stressful event rather than triggered by ongoing anxiety. Panic attacks are short-lived (5–20 minutes), but are unpleasant and frightening experiences, involving a rush of intense psychological and physical conditions. A person having a panic attack may experience overwhelming fear and anxiety, plus other symptoms, such as dizziness, shortness of breath, nausea, trembling, sweating, rapid heartbeat, chest pain and confusion. Although the symptoms are scary, panic attacks are not in themselves physically harmful. People with a panic disorder experience recurring feelings of anxiety, stress and panic on a regular basis, inducing more panic attacks, often for no reason. It affects roughly 2 in 100 people in the UK and is more common in women. The frequency of panic attacks can be from once or twice a month to several times a week, leading to ongoing feelings of worry in anticipation of the next attack. Panic disorder often begins in people aged between 20 and 35 and is thought to be rare in older age groups, although older people can and do experience panic attacks, usually due to life changes, such as the death of a spouse, health issues and depression. All people with panic disorder will get panic attacks on a recurring basis. Some people have attacks once or twice a month, while others have them several times a week. But simply having panic attacks does not necessarily mean your relative has a panic disorder.

Try not to let the fear of a panic attack control your relative and importantly, remind them that panic attacks always pass and that their fears are caused by anxiety so they should try to ride out the attack. Confronting their fears lets them discover that nothing bad is going to happen. If you are with them, you can provide reassurance. Breathing exercises and practicing mindfulness can also be very helpful in managing anxiety (see pages 131–133 for more details). However, it is very important to seek medical help if their panic attacks become more frequent.

If you are concerned about your relative's anxiety, then the first port of call should be a chat with their GP to rule out any unknown physical cause of the anxiety. There are anti-anxiety medications which can help, but they may also suggest regular exercise, a referral for counselling, or contacting a support group. Caregivers are clearly an important source of support and can help by learning about the condition, providing reassurance and maintaining a normal routine. Fortunately, there are a number of organisations and charities who provide great support for those who suffer with panic attacks. Support groups are a way for them to share common experiences and provide tips on how to cope.

For further help and information, contact Anxiety UK at www.anxietyuk.org.uk, or No Panic at www.nopanic.org.uk. MIND also has helpful tips on anxiety. Visit www.mind.org.uk.

Depression

Many issues can cause depression as people age, such as retirement, the death of friends and loved ones, increased isolation, or medical problems. Left untreated, depression can impact on physical health, impair memory and concentration, and prevent people from enjoying life. The symptoms of depression can affect all aspects of life, including energy, appetite, sleep and interest in work, hobbies and relationships. Many depressed older people, or their relatives, fail to recognise the symptoms of depression and/or do not take the steps to get the help they need. There can be an assumption that older people have good reason to be down, or that depression is just part of getting older. Older people may be reluctant to talk about their feelings, or to ask for help, or they may simply be frightened of admitting to depression. It is so important to remember that depression is not a sign of weakness, or a character flaw. It can happen to anyone, at any age, no matter what your background, or your previous accomplishments in life.

As people grow older, they face significant life changes that can put them at risk of depression. Causes and risk factors that contribute to depression in older adults and the elderly include illness and disability, chronic or severe pain, cognitive decline and damage to body image due to surgery, or disease. Living alone and having a dwindling social circle, due to deaths or relocation, as well as decreased mobility, due to illness or loss of driving privileges, can also lead to depression. Sufferers may feel a lack of purposelessness, or loss of identity. Fear of death or dying, or anxiety over financial problems or health issues can cause depression, as can the death of friends, family members, pets or the loss of a spouse or partner.

As we age, we tend to experience more loss and this is painful. The loss can be felt in different ways, as a loss of independence, or of mobility, health, your long-time career, or someone you love. Grieving over these losses is normal and healthy, even if the feelings of sadness last for a long time. Losing all hope and joy, however, is not normal. Distinguishing between grief and clinical depression is not always easy, since they share many of the same symptoms. However, there are ways to tell the difference. Grief involves a wide variety of emotions and a mix of good and bad days. Even in the middle of the grieving process, there will be moments of pleasure or happiness, but with depression, the feelings of emptiness and despair are constant. Signs include feelings of guilt, suicidal thoughts, or a preoccupation with dying, feelings of hopelessness or worthlessness, slow speech and body movements, the inability to function at work or home and sometimes, seeing or hearing imaginary things.

Symptoms of depression can also occur as part of medical problems such as dementia, or as a side effect of prescription drugs. Medical conditions which can cause depression include Parkinson's disease, stroke, heart disease, cancer, diabetes, thyroid disorders, vitamin B12 deficiency, dementia and Alzheimer's disease, lupus and multiple sclerosis. Symptoms of depression can also be a side effect of many commonly prescribed drugs and especially a combination of many drugs taken together. Older adults are more sensitive because, as we age, our bodies become less efficient at metabolising and processing drugs. Medications that can cause or worsen depression include blood pressure medication, beta-blockers, sleeping pills, tranquillisers, medication for Parkinson's disease, ulcer medication, heart drugs, steroids, high-cholesterol and painkillers and arthritis drugs. Alcohol can make symptoms of depression, irritability and anxiety worse and impairs brain function. Alcohol interacts in negative ways with numerous medications, including antidepressants, and affects quality of sleep.

Signs of depression include overriding sadness, constant fatigue, abandoning or losing interest in hobbies or other pastimes, a reluctance to be with friends, engage in activities or to leave the house, weight loss or loss of appetite, sleep disturbances, anxiety, increased use of alcohol or other drugs, suicidal thoughts or attempts, aggravated aches and pains, memory problems, lack of energy, slowed movement and speech and irritability. The more active people are, physically, mentally, and socially, the better they will feel. Physical activity has powerful mood-boosting effects. In fact, research suggests it may be just as effective as antidepressants in relieving depression. The best part is that the benefits come without side effects. Encourage walking, taking the stairs, or if mobility is more difficult, suggest seated exercises, such as leg and arm lifts and circles. Try to encourage older people to socialise with others, or talk on the phone. They must also try to get enough sleep and maintain a healthy diet. Encourage your relative to get out and about by volunteering, taking up a new hobby, or looking after a pet (see pages 133–135).

Antidepressants should be used with care if prescribed by the GP. Older adults are more sensitive to drug side effects and vulnerable to interactions with other medicines they may be taking. Recent studies have also found that drugs, such as Prozac, can cause rapid bone density loss and therefore, a higher risk of fractures and falls. Because of these safety concerns, older adults on antidepressants should be carefully monitored. Your relative can also try herbal remedies, acupuncture and natural supplements, which can be effective in treating depression, and in most cases, are much safer for older adults than antidepressants (see pages 129–130 for details on acupuncture). Omega-3 fatty acids may boost the effectiveness of antidepressants, or work as a standalone treatment for depression. St John's Wort can help with mild or moderate symptoms of depression, but should not be taken in conjunction with antidepressants. Folic acid can help relieve the symptoms of depression when combined with other treatments.

Therapy works well on depression, because it addresses the underlying causes of the depression, rather than just the symptoms. It can ease loneliness and the hopelessness of depression. Therapy helps people work through stressful life changes, heal losses, process difficult emotions, change negative thinking patterns and develop better coping skills. Support groups for depression, illness, or bereavement are a safe place to share experiences, advice, and encouragement. Cognitive behavioural therapy (CBT) is often used to treat depression and focuses very much on the symptoms, rather than the underlying causes of depression.

If an older person you care about is depressed, you can make a difference by offering emotional support. Listen with patience and compassion. Try not to criticise the feelings they express, but point out realities and offer hope. You can also help by making sure that you get an accurate diagnosis and appropriate treatment. Go with them to appointments and offer moral support. Take them out, as depression is less likely when minds remain active. Suggest activities to do together, such as walks, attending an art class, taking a trip to a museum or going to the cinema. Group outings, visits from friends and family members, or trips to the local senior or community centre can help combat isolation and loneliness. Be gently insistent if your plans are refused, because depressed people often feel better when they're around others, even when they do not think they will.

Plan and prepare healthy meals. A poor diet can make depression worse, so make sure your loved one is eating well, with plenty of fruit, vegetables, whole grains and some protein at every meal. Make sure all medications are taken as instructed and watch for suicidal tendencies. If you are worried, see their GP.

MIND has helpful information on depression. Visit www.mind.org.uk.

Insomnia

Everyone has a bad night's sleep occasionally, but for some, insomnia is a serious issue, which can have serious consequences. Insomnia is more common in older people and is often debilitating as it can go on for days, months or even years. If normal sleep patterns are disrupted, it can affect memory and cause depression, anxiety, irritability and many other problems.

Sleep requirements change with age. Babies sleep for about 16 hours out of every 24, adolescents need 9 hours and adults need between 7 and 9 hours each night. As we age, however, we often wake earlier and go to sleep earlier. Quality of sleep is as important as quantity.

Older people tend to sleep less deeply and for less time. There are also two types of insomnia: the inability to get to sleep and inability to stay asleep. Insomnia can be caused by stress due to work, bereavement, divorce, moving house and many other issues which have an effect on overworking the mind, so that you cannot switch off. Poor sleep hygiene, such as the wrong temperature, uncomfortable bedding and too much light, can all affect your relative's ability to get to sleep and to stay asleep. An irregular sleeping routine can affect their ability to fall asleep, as can stimulants, such as coffee, tea, chocolate and smoking. Alcohol initially promotes sleep, but later fragments it. As we age, the brain's internal clock shifts to an earlier sleep cycle, so older people tend to fall asleep earlier, but wake earlier and night-time sleeping can also be affected if naps are taken during the day.

Medication can have significant effects on sleeping, particularly if your relative is taking multiple prescriptions. Pain and physical discomfort will also inhibit sleep. As we age, we need to go to the toilet more often during the night, which wakes us as well. And if your partner snores, it will definitely affect your sleep! Try to encourage your relative to get into a good routine with a regular time to sleep and wake up. Exercising during the day, preferably in the morning, will help, and it is best to avoid exercise for a few hours before bed. Make sure your relative's bedroom is dark enough, that the bed and bedding is comfortable and that the room is not too hot or too cold. Try to encourage them to make time to take a warm bath or shower before bed to relax. They should avoid heavy meals, caffeine, smoking and alcohol for at least three hours before bed, and try not to sleep or nap during the day. Watching television in bed, or using phones or tablets, can prevent the mind from switching off, so limit their use before bed. They should also try to avoid sleeping pills and never take them without advice from their GP. Mindfulness can be very effective to calm the mind before bed (see pages 131–133 for details) and sometimes, counting sheep really can help!

Huntington's disease (HD)

Huntington's disease is an inherited condition, causing progressive brain damage. The disease is caused by a faulty gene, which creates a protein which damages and ultimately kills off brain cells. As the disease progresses, it leads to depression and psychiatric problems, uncontrolled movement, problems with eating and swallowing, behavioural changes, memory loss and poor cognition. Around 12 people out of every 100,000 in the UK have Huntington's. The disease affects both men and women and it is possible to develop it at any age. Typically, most people who develop problems are diagnosed between 35 and 55 years old. The condition generally progresses for around 10–25 years.

Although symptoms of HD can vary, the progression of the disease is fairly predictable. Early symptoms, such as personality changes, mood swings and unusual behaviour, are often subtle and can be overlooked. Patients can often alternate between excitement and apathy, and between depression and excitement. A general lack of coordination becomes more apparent. Patients can be unsteady on their feet and develop jerky body movements. Loss of motor control can make eating and swallowing difficult. Behavioural changes become more pronounced and there is a gradual decline in communication and mental abilities. Some patients may develop dementia. Although a genetic test for HD has been available for those with a family history of the disease since the early 1990s, some people prefer not to know if they are carriers. However, finding out may give them more time to get appropriate treatment and come to terms with the disease.

Unfortunately, there is no cure as yet for Huntington's, but research continues worldwide. In the meantime, some aspects of the disease can be managed successfully with medication, specialist therapies and keeping as active as possible. Medication may be prescribed to control involuntary movements, depression and mood swings. Speech therapy can help with communication and swallowing issues and physiotherapy can help maintain balance and mobility. Local authority social services can provide occupational therapy to help make daily living much easier with home adaptations and equipment (see pages 70–73 for more information on care assessments). As well as your relative's GP and local social services, there are some organisations which offer specialist advice and support.

You can contact The Huntington's Disease Association (HDA) on their website at www.hda.org.uk, or there is more information on the NHS website at www.nhs.uk/conditions/huntingtons-disease.

CHAPTER TEN

End of Life Care

End of life care supports those people who are in the last months of their life. It is a difficult time for those about to leave us and for the people caring for them, but it is important to provide the best possible care and to enable our loved ones to die with dignity.

Health professionals assisting you with end of life care should ensure that they ask about your relative's preferences and express wishes and incorporate these as much as possible into their care. They should also support the family and other carers.

Palliative care

Palliative care focuses on helping people to maintain the best possible quality of life and aims to prevent and alleviate the symptoms of illness for them when curative treatment is no longer possible. It should also address the wider emotional, social and practical needs of people as they near the end of their life. Such care can be delivered in hospitals and hospices, via community services, or at home. Support also extends to family and friends, who may have concerns about the person and their illness. Palliative care can be given at the same time as other treatments, such as chemotherapy or radiotherapy.

Having a terminal illness is very difficult for both the patient and family to manage. Feelings can change from day-to-day, hour-to-hour and even minute-to-minute. It is common for people to feel denial, anger, fear, depression and even guilt, often all at the same time. Supporting and caring for someone with a terminal illness may be too much for you to handle by yourself. Try to talk to others about your feelings and how you are coping as this can help you to deal with your emotions and the impact the illness is having on your life. You may find it easier to talk to a close friend, rather than to someone in the family, because this means you can be yourself and express yourself more easily, without the complications of family issues getting in the way. Alternatively, you may find it helpful to speak to a counsellor, or to someone at a support group. Providing care for someone who is ill can place great physical and emotional demands on you and it is important that you take time out to recharge by spending time with your friends, or having some time alone if you feel tired or overwhelmed. Losing a relative is tough and a life-changing experience, so do not be too hard on yourself. Feeling guilty is common, but remember that you can only do your best. You may also feel a need to express your anger. This is normal. Writing things down can be very helpful, as even with members of your family or close friends, it can be difficult to express your feelings fully. A hobby or a form of sport can also help to release your anger and frustration.

The person you are caring for could be, and is most likely to, feel the same way. Try to talk to them about it and learn what is frightening you and them. Ask questions of the professionals treating your relative as knowing the facts will often help. However, denial is a common coping mechanism that both patient and carer will often use when the person is diagnosed with a terminal illness. If you are in denial about the situation regarding your relative's health, do not blame yourself, or feel that you must do something about your feelings. The person you are caring for is very likely to have mood swings and good and bad days. They may even try to hide their feelings from you, or behave in a way that you do not expect. You may find they change from not wanting to upset you by talking about their illness to blaming you for it. Other times, they may act as if nothing is bothering them. This can be very distressing for you and may affect your relationship with the person you are caring for. Be honest and talk about all your feelings, not just the positive ones. Bad days are to be expected, so you do not need to pretend to be cheerful when you are not as this can stop you and your relative who is ill talking about the things that are important to you both while you still have the opportunity. Some terminal illnesses, including dementia, can have an effect on the person's personality and lead to them having sudden fits of anger. Talk to your GP, or another healthcare professional, about this.

My father had never hit me in his life, but towards the end, in the hospice one day, he reached out and tried to smack me as I walked past. He had no strength and it barely registered, but I was very surprised and upset nonetheless.

'Did you just try to smack me?' I asked him.

He just glared back at me, clearly so angry and frustrated to be stuck in his failing body and mind. I went over and gave him a hug and then I left the room for a minute to have a little cry. Afterwards, I was able to rationalise this as part of his dementia and even smile about it years later, but it is still upsetting to think about how much this disease changed my father and how it affected his quality of life in his last few years and the relationship with us, his family.

Hospices

The driving force behind hospice, or palliative, care is the desire to transform the experience of dying and to make it as kind as possible. Even in the 21st century, too many people die in avoidable pain and distress. In hospices, multi-disciplinary teams strive to offer freedom from pain, dignity, peace and calm at the end of life. Underpinning this care is a philosophy that takes as its starting point the affirmation of death as a natural part of life. Built on that bedrock are the values of respect, choice, empowerment, holistic care and compassion. Hospices care for the whole person, aiming to meet all needs:

physical, emotional, social and spiritual. They care for the person who is dying, and for those who love them: at home, in day care and in the hospice. Nearly half of all people admitted to a hospice return home again. The average length of stay is just 13 days. All care is free of charge. Within hospices, you will find a range of services, including pain control, symptom relief, skilled nursing care, counselling, complementary therapies, spiritual care, art, music, physiotherapy, reminiscence, beauty treatments and bereavement support. Staff and volunteers work in multi-professional teams to provide care based on individual need and personal choice.

There are also trained palliative care doctors and nurses within the NHS, who will help care for your relative in hospital or at home.

You can find useful information on end of life care on the NHS website at www.nhs.uk/conditions/end-of-life-care and at Dying Matters, www.dyingmatters.org.

Coping with bereavement

At some point, most of us will suffer the death of someone we love. Yet day-to-day, we do not think and talk about death as we encounter it less often than our grand-relatives did. For them, the death of a brother or sister, friend or relative was a common experience in their childhood or teenage years. For us, these losses usually happen much later in life, so we do not have much of a chance either to learn about grieving – how it feels, the right things to do and say – nor do we know how to come to terms with it.

Grief is felt after any sort of loss, but most powerfully, after the death of someone we love. It is not just one feeling, but a whole succession of feelings and it takes a while to work through it. Usually, we grieve the most for someone that we have known for some time. In the few hours, or days following the death of a close relative or friend, most people feel shocked, as though they cannot believe it has actually happened. They may feel like this even if the death has been expected. This sense of emotional numbness can be a help in getting through all the important practical arrangements that have to be made, such as getting in touch with relatives and organising the funeral. However, this feeling of unreality may become a problem if it goes on too long. Seeing the body of the dead person may, for some, be an important way of beginning to overcome this. Similarly, for many people, the funeral or memorial service is an occasion when the reality of what has happened really starts to sink in. It may be distressing to see the body, or attend the funeral, but these are important parts of the process of saying goodbye to those we love.

When the numbness disappears, it can be replaced by a dreadful sense of agitation and yearning for the dead person. There can be a feeling of wanting somehow to find them, even though this is clearly impossible. This can make it difficult to relax, concentrate, or to sleep properly. Dreams can be very upsetting. Some people feel that they see their loved one everywhere they go. People often feel very angry after bereavement. Sometimes, this anger is directed towards the doctors and nurses who did not prevent the death, towards friends and relatives who did not do enough, or even towards the person who has, by dying, left them.

Guilt is another common feeling. People find themselves going over in their minds all the things they would have liked to have said or done. They may even consider what they could have done differently, or other actions that might have prevented the death. Of course, death is usually beyond anyone's control and a bereaved person may need to be reminded of this. Some people may feel guilty if they feel relieved that their loved one has died after a painful or distressing illness. This feeling of relief is natural, understandable and very common. You should not feel guilty about feeling this way.

This state of agitation is usually strongest about two weeks after the death, but is soon followed by times of quiet sadness or depression, withdrawal and silence. These sudden changes of emotion can be confusing to friends or relatives, but are part of the normal process of grief. Depression can become more frequent as the agitation stage lessens – often four to six weeks later. Spasms of grief can occur at any time, sparked off by people, places or things that bring back memories of the dead person. During this time, it may appear to others as though the bereaved person is spending a great deal of time just sitting, doing nothing. In fact, they are usually thinking about the person they have lost, going over again and again both the good and bad times they had together. This is a quiet, but essential part of coming to terms with the death.

Eventually, the fierce pain of early bereavement begins to fade. The depression reduces and it is possible to think about other things and think about the future. However, the sense of having lost a part of oneself never goes away entirely. For bereaved partners, there are constant reminders of their new singleness, in seeing other couples together and from the deluge of media images of happy families.

Letting go is the final phase of grieving. The depression clears, sleep improves and energy returns to normal. Sexual feelings which may have vanished now return. Remember, there is no standard way of grieving, everyone copes differently. And it is important to remember that. Ask for help with bereavement from your GP. If lack of sleep becomes a serious problem, the doctor may prescribe a short-term supply of sleeping tablets. Your GP can also arrange for counselling, or can advise on support groups for bereavement. They may prescribe antidepressants if symptoms are severe, or refer you for further help from a specialist.

Helping a bereaved relative

When your relative is bereaved, whether their partner's death was sudden, or prolonged, it takes a long time for them to adjust to living alone. When people have lived together for many years and shared the day-to-day responsibilities of running a home, it can be very difficult to develop new routines and to have the basic confidence to continue as one person rather than two. Having to take on new and additional tasks can be daunting, but there are things you can do to assist your relative to adjust.

Help them to make a list of everything that needs doing at home. This includes bills which need paying, regular essential shopping requirements, gardening, rubbish collection and keeping essential appointments. Help them to decide what their priorities should be from this list and then agree what needs to be done daily, weekly, monthly and so on. You can then help them to put a schedule together of what to do when. If the workload seems too daunting, try to suggest to them that they get some help at home, either temporarily or permanently, if needed. Setting up direct debit payments can be a great help, so that they do not need to worry about organising to pay regular bills. You can also help them with much of their admin, especially if you have agreed Power of Attorney (see pages 36–40 for more information).

Adjusting to life on your own has its ups and downs and it is important to encourage your relative to express their feelings in order to come to terms with loss. Talking can help, but they should not feel pressured into it. Family and friends are a natural source of emotional support, but may not always be readily available, or your relative may prefer to speak to someone who is uninvolved, such as their GP, who can advise them on how to deal with the symptoms of grief, such as sleeplessness, anxiety or depression. The GP may offer counselling, or prescribe medication, if symptoms do not improve. Professional counselling can help your relative to express their emotions, which may be more complicated than simply missing the person lost. It can be a good way to explore feelings and to come closer to some sort of resolution. Websites and forums can also provide an anonymous place for your relative to say what they really feel in total freedom and it can be a great help to speak to people who have shared similar experiences.

You can also help someone who is bereaved to start socialising again. If they are nervous or reluctant, ask them what they have done in the past that they would like to do again, or whether there are some activities they have never done, but would like to try. Maybe they can take up a new hobby (see pages 135–141 for suggestions) which can be interesting and a great way to meet new people, or study simply for the pleasure of knowing something new (see page 92 for ideas.) Maybe they can think about volunteering (see pages 140–141) or get into exercising (see pages 118–123). If they are used to going on an annual holiday, or taking day trips with their partner, they may feel nervous about travelling on their own, but perhaps they can arrange to travel with a friend, or there may be local community groups organising coach tours or train trips. There are also many companies arranging holidays for older single travellers. Travel agents can help, or you can search online (see pages 142–143 for more advice). They may also want to consider getting a pet. If your relative can cope with a pet and likes animals, they can provide untold levels of love and companionship (see pages 133–135).

Making sure that your relative eats healthily for one is really important. Often, they may think there is little point in cooking for one, but if they do not eat well, their energy levels and physical and emotional health will suffer. They should be encouraged to start the day with a good breakfast, such as fruit juice and wholegrain cereal with milk, or eggs on toast.

Top tip: Help your relative to plan meals ahead and make batches of food for them to keep in the freezer. Soups and pasta are great for this.

A sandwich made with wholegrain bread, a savoury filling, tomato and lettuce can be just as nourishing as a cooked meal, if they do not feel like cooking. You can order food for them through supermarkets who offer online delivery, so they do not need to worry about shopping. If you help them to get online, they can do internet food shopping for themselves, if they wish. (For more information on technology see page 98.)

How to register a death

After someone dies, you have five days to register their death. You should register the death at the registry office local to where the person died, so that the documents can be processed as quickly as possible. Details of your local registry office can be found in your local phone book, or online at www.gov.uk.

- It takes about 30 minutes to register a death. Make sure you ask for as many copies of the death certificate as you think you might need to notify the bank, solicitor and other authorities. Often these companies will not accept photocopies. You have to pay for these copies
- You should register the death with the Tell Us Once service online at www.gov.uk, which will notify all the main parties for you, including:
  - HM Revenue and Customs (HMRC) – to deal with personal tax (you need to contact HMRC separately for business taxes, like VAT)
  - Department for Work and Pensions (DWP) – to cancel benefits, for example, Income Support
  - Passport Office – to cancel a British passport
  - Driver and Vehicle Licensing Agency (DVLA) – to cancel a licence and remove the person as the keeper of up to five vehicles (contact DVLA separately if you keep or sell a vehicle)
  - The local council – to cancel Housing Benefit, Council Tax Benefit, a Blue Badge, inform council housing services and remove the person from the electoral register
  - Veterans UK – to cancel Armed Forces Compensation Scheme payments.

HM Revenue and Customs (HMRC) and the Department for Work and Pensions (DWP) will contact you about the tax, benefits and entitlements of the person who died.

Tell Us Once will also contact some public sector pension schemes so that they cancel future pension payments. They will notify:

- My Civil Service Pension
- NHS Pension Scheme
- Armed Forces Pension Scheme
- Pension schemes for NHS staff, teachers, police and firefighters in Scotland
- Local authority pension schemes, except where Tell Us Once is not available.

Top tip: Always get more copies of the death certificate than the registry office suggests, as you always need more than they recommend. Between eight to 10 copies is normally enough.

If the person died in a house or hospital, the death is usually registered by a relative. The registrar would normally only allow other people to register if there are no relatives available. In this case, it could be someone who witnessed the death – a hospital official, or a person making funeral arrangements. You will need various documents and information to register a death, including the medical certificate of the cause of death, signed by a doctor, and if possible, the deceased's birth certificate, marriage or civil partnership certificate and/or NHS Medical Card. You must tell the registrar the deceased person's full name at time of death, any names previously used, including maiden surname, the person's date and place of birth (town and county if born in the UK, and country if born abroad), their last address, their occupation, the full name, date of birth and occupation of a surviving spouse or civil partner and notify them if they were getting a state pension, or any other state benefit.

The registrar will give you – as long as there is no post-mortem – a certificate for burial or cremation (called the green form), which gives permission for the body to be buried, or for the application to apply for the body to be cremated, a certificate of registration of death (form BD8), issued for social security purposes if the person was on a state pension or benefits (read the information on the back, complete and return it, if it applies) and you should also receive a booklet called 'What to do after a death', which contains advice on wills, funerals and financial help. You may need to tell a number of different government departments and agencies about the death. The registrar can advise you on how to go about this. If a post-mortem is needed, the coroner will issue any documents you need as quickly as possible after its completion. Where the cause of death is unclear, sudden or suspicious, the doctor, hospital or registrar will report the death to the coroner. The coroner must then decide if there should be further investigation. The registrar cannot register the death until the coroner's decision has been made.

You can find more details on registering a death at www.gov.uk.

Arranging a funeral

Because most people tend to avoid the subject of death and funerals, they tend to be generally poorly equipped to make informed decisions when they are bereaved. Consequently, myths abound and most people do not shop around, or question the quotes or advice they receive. Beyond the basic decision of burial or cremation, people may need to consider the technicalities and pitfalls of options, such as body donation, burial on private land or at sea.

For those planning ahead, they need to be aware of the costs of making the wrong person the executor of their will, the possible benefits of appointing a power of attorney over their financial and health affairs and why they might consider making an advance decision (see pages 36–42 for further details).

Many people are worried about the cost of a funeral. The average, basic funeral in the UK now starts at about £3000. However, there are alternatives. There are many independent funeral directors who offer a direct cremation or burial service. This pares funerals down to absolute basics and entails the deceased being collected, placed in a standard coffin and cremated at the funeral director's convenience and choice of crematorium, usually without ceremony. This suits families who want to separate the ceremony from the disposal of the body, by having a memorial service on another day, for example, or those who simply have no one, or want no one, to attend. It gets away from the normal, black funeral and its related expenses. The cost of this direct type of funeral is usually between £995–£1700, depending on location. This price includes all fees.

You can decide to organise a burial or cremation yourself if you prefer. Some families decide to keep the deceased at home and possibly even bury them on their own land. Of course, these funerals are, in effect, free. Common myths include that there is some law stating that you have to use a funeral director, bodies and coffins have to be transported in a hearse, that you have to be embalmed to be viewed, that cremated remains are mixed together and that coffins are reused. None of these are true.

If you do use a funeral firm, choosing one can be difficult, especially if you are confronted with having to make a quick decision. Membership of a reputable trade association should be mandatory. By choosing a funeral firm which is a member of the National Association of Funeral Directors, you can be assured it is quality assessed and can be expected to provide a guaranteed level of service. Member firms are bound by a code of practice against which their performance can be measured. In the sad event that the experience is not all that it could be, you can contact the Funeral Arbitration Scheme. To search for a member firm, use the NAFD member search at www.nafd.org.uk. Many people ask friends or relatives to recommend a firm that they have dealt with, or have heard positive comments about. If you do not have the opportunity to ask advice from others, your local solicitors, or GP surgery, will know of local funeral firms. Failing that, you can research firms in your area by browsing the internet, or looking for advertisements in your local newspapers or telephone directories.

You can change your mind about funeral arrangements. If you have signed an agreement for services to be provided, this may not be straightforward, but members of the NAFD should always withdraw in favour of another funeral firm under these circumstances. You should be aware, however, that there may be costs incurred with the first company and you will be responsible for paying their bill. If the funeral arrangements were made in a place other than the funeral firm's own offices, the transaction is covered under the home selling regulations set out by the Consumer Protection Act 2009. In these circumstances, you have seven days from the moment you enter into the contract with the funeral firm to cancel and instruct another. Cancellation must be in writing. Again, there may be costs incurred prior to cancellation that must be paid. For example, if you have already asked a funeral firm to transfer the deceased to their premises, you can still use a different firm to deal with the funeral arrangements. The company you contact to deal with the funeral will arrange for the transfer of the deceased to their premises. However, it will still be necessary for you to pay the other firm for the removal of the deceased.

Planning ahead for a funeral can make financial sense, but paying for funerals in advance is another area that can be complicated. Generally speaking, insurance-based products can be expensive in the long run and may not cover the cost of a funeral, especially if your relative lives for longer than they think. The small print may reveal that any failure with monthly payments will result in the policy being void. Shopping around is very important. Undertakers vary hugely in how they operate, who really owns them, how flexible they are and how much they charge.

Conclusion

As I mentioned in my introduction to this book, I have tried to pull together as much information as I can to help family carers look after older relatives, in order to help you to find some of the answers to questions you may have, and to help reduce the stress of caring just a little. So many more of us will take on caring responsibilities over the next few decades, as our populations continue to age.

Everyone ages differently, at different ages and with different physical and mental health challenges to confront. All families have their own personal dynamics and relationships vary from very close to quite distant. Consequently, no single volume can offer up solutions to every individual challenge older people and their family carers may face. However, I hope that you have found that this book can provide some level of support for you, both practically and emotionally.

Being a carer is hard work, because you do exactly that – you care. You are required to source not only practical solutions to problems, but also to provide essential emotional support. Let me reassure you … you really are doing the best you can, and that's all you can do. Feeling stressed and guilty at times is inevitable, but it will not help you get through the minefield of elder care and it may even cause you to compromise your own health.

If I have achieved nothing else with this manual, I have at least provided my own two sons with a guide as to what to do with me as I age. I wish them good luck – I probably won't be easy!

A–Z of Care Jargon

When you have to start dealing with the problems associated with old age, there is a great deal of terminology which is often hard to understand. Here are some of the key terms explained:

Advanced Decision/Living Will: An Advanced Decision, also known as a Living Will, is a statement explaining what medical treatment the individual would not want in the future, should that individual 'lack capacity', as defined by the Mental Capacity Act 2005.

Assistive technology: Assistive technology (AT) is a generic term that includes assistive, adaptive, and rehabilitative devices for people with disabilities.

Care assessments: An assessment which looks at your relative's needs and recommends the appropriate services. Normally, an assessment is required before any services can be provided by the social services department of a local authority, but if the need is urgent, the local authority can provide help without carrying out the assessment.

Care home: A care home is a residential setting, where a number of older people live, usually in single rooms, and has access to on-site care services. Since April 2002, all homes in England, Scotland and Wales are known as 'care homes', but are registered to provide different levels of care. A home registered simply as a care home will provide personal care only, i.e. help with washing, dressing and giving medication. A home registered as a care home with nursing will provide the same personal care, but also have a qualified nurse on duty 24 hours a day to carry out nursing tasks. These homes are for people who are physically or mentally frail, or those who need regular attention from a nurse. Other homes will provide specific dementia care.

Carer's assessment: Unpaid carers are entitled to an assessment of their own needs, if they are providing, or intending to provide, a substantial amount of care on a regular basis. If you, as a carer, have your own need for community care services because of ill health or disability, you may also be eligible for your own community care assessment.

Dementia: The word dementia is used to describe a group of symptoms. Although dementia is commonly thought of as memory loss, the reality is much more complex and symptoms between the different forms of dementia can vary a great deal. Dementia symptoms can include memory loss, confusion and mood changes.

NHS Continuing Care: This is a package of continuing care provided outside hospital. If your relative is eligible, they can receive NHS Continuing Healthcare in any setting – for example, in their own home. The NHS will pay for care home fees, including board and accommodation or for care requirements at home. NHS Continuing Care is free, unlike social and community care services provided by local authorities, for which a charge may be made, depending on your relative's income and savings.

Palliative Care: This focuses on relieving and preventing the suffering of patients living with chronic diseases, as well as patients who are nearing the end of life.

Personal Budgets: Personalisation, also known as self-directed support, is a way of working that gives people and their carers more control, choice and flexibility over how they plan and manage their social care support.

Personal Care Plans: A personal care plan informs carers about your relative and sets out the key things your relative does and does not like and also specifies the little things which can make a big difference. Setting out a personal care plan can be helpful if you are bringing carers into your relative's home, or if they are going into a care home.

Power of Attorney: Power of Attorney enables an older person to give power to another person to look after their affairs when they no longer have capacity to do so themselves – for example, if they have a stroke, develop dementia or any other illness which impairs their ability to make decisions. There are two types of Power of Attorney: Property and Finance and Health and Wellbeing.

Probate: A Grant of Probate is an order of the court, giving one or more people the legal authority to administer the estate of a deceased person, in order to distribute it correctly to the beneficiaries.

State pension: This provides a regular income once a person reaches state pension age. It is based on National Insurance contributions and the amount you get depends on how much you paid in.

Stroke: A stroke is a brain attack. It happens when the blood supply to part of your brain is cut off and brain cells are damaged or die, caused by a clot or bleeding in the brain.

Trusts: Trusts are there to provide income to others in specific circumstances, either within a person's lifetime or after their death.

Wills: A will ensures that those people who your relative wants to benefit from their estate on death receive their entitlement. These could be relatives, friends or charities.

Contacts

Remember, some numbers may charge you for your call, depending on your phone tariff.

Action on Elder Abuse
Report abuse of older people.
080 8808 8141
www.elderabuse.org.uk

Age UK
General help and advice for older people.
0800 678 1602
www.ageuk.org.uk

Arthritis Care
Help for those with arthritis.
0300 790 0400
www.arthritiscare.org.uk

Beat
Help with anorexia and eating disorders.
0808 801 0677
www.beateatingdisorders.org.uk

Bladder & Bowel
Advice on bladder and bowel problems.
0161 607 8200
www.bbuk.org.uk
See also:
www.bowelcanceruk.org.uk

Blue Badge
Register for disabled parking.
www.gov.uk/get-blue-badge

British Acupuncture Council
Find an acupuncturist.
020 8735 0400
www.acupuncture.org.uk

British Association of Dermatologists
Find a dermatologist.
0207 383 0266
www.bad.org.uk

British Dental Association
Find a dentist.
020 7935 0875
www.bda.org

British Heart Foundation
Information about the heart and heart disease.
0300 330 3311
Mon–Fri 9 a.m.–5 p.m.
www.bhf.org.uk

British Gas/Homecare
If you are a Homecare customer, they will come out within the day to fix heating problems. Make sure you tell them if your relative is older or alone, to prioritise your call out.
0333 200 8899
Mon–Fri 8 a.m.–8 p.m.; Sat 9 a.m.–5 p.m.
www.britishgas.co.uk/home-services

British Red Cross
First Aid courses.
0344 871 11 11
www.redcross.org.uk

Care Quality Commission
The Commission ranks and rates all care homes and GPs in the UK.
03000 616161
www.cqc.org.uk

Chartered Society of Physiotherapy
Find a physiotherapist.
020 7306 6666
ww.csp.org.uk

Citizens Advice
Offers advice on consumer rights and help with complaints and refunds.
03444 111 444
03444 77 20 20 (Wales)
Mon–Fri 9 a.m.–5 p.m.
www.citizensadvice.org.uk

Dementia/Alzheimer's
Information about dementia and Alzheimer's.
0800 888 6678
020 8036 5400
0300 222 1122
www.dementiauk.org
www.alzheimers.org.uk

Department for Work and Pensions (DWP)
Advice and support on pensions and benefits.
www.gov.uk/government/organisations/department-for-work-pensions

Diabetes UK
Information about diabetes.
0345 123 2399
www.diabetes.org.uk

Disability Holidays Guide
Help with holidays and travel.
0345 3000 250 (Railcard)
www.disabilityholidaysguide.com

Doro
Mobile phones designed for older people.
0800 026 5479
8 a.m.–7 p.m.
www.doro.com/en-gb

Dying Matters
Help with bereavement.
0800 021 4466
www.dyingmatters.org

English Heritage
Visit historic houses and gardens.
0370 333 1181
www.english-heritage.org.uk

Find Your Local Authority
www.gov.uk/find-local-council

General Optical Council
Find an optician.
020 7580 3898
www.optical.org

HMRC
Advice on all aspects of tax.
www.gov.uk/government/organisations/hm-revenue-customs

Hospice UK
Find a hospice.
020 7520 8200
www.hospiceuk.org

Institute of Financial Accountants (IFA)
Find an accountant in the UK.
0203 567 5999
https://ifa.org.uk

The Law Society
Find a UK solicitor.
020 7242 1222
www.lawsociety.org.uk

Milk & More
Milk and groceries delivered to your door by a milkman.
0345 606 3606
9 a.m.–4.30 p.m.
www.milkandmore.co.uk

MIND
Help and support for mental health issues.
020 8519 2122
www.mind.org.uk

The Money Advice Service
Advice on personal finances and money matters.
0800 138 7777
8 a.m.–5 p.m.
www.moneyadviceservice.org.uk

National Trust
Visit historic houses and gardens.
0344 800 1895
www.nationaltrust.org.uk

NHS Direct
Helpful health advice by phone and online.
111 is the NHS non-emergency number. It's fast, easy and free.
www.nhsdirect.nhs.uk

NI Direct
Advice on money, pensions, motoring and more.
www.nidirect.gov.uk

Ofcom Nuisance Call Complaints
Help with tackling nuisance calls and messages.

020 7981 3040
www.ofcom.org.uk/phones-telecoms-and-internet/advice-for-consumers/problems/tackling-nuisance-calls-and-messages

Ombudsman
Help to resolve complaints between consumers and companies, including care homes and energy providers.
www.ombudsman-services.org

Osteopathy
Find a UK osteopath.
020 7357 6655
www.osteopathy.org.uk

Parkinson's UK
Advice on Parkinson's disease
0808 800 0303
www.parkinsons.org.uk

The Pension Advisory Service (TPAS)
Free information, advice and guidance on personal pensions.
0800 011 3797
Mon–Fri 9 a.m.–5 p.m.
www.pensionsadvisoryservice.org.uk (web chat available)

Pension wise
0800 138 3944
Mon–Fri 8 a.m.–8 p.m.
www.pensionwise.gov.uk

Revitalise
Respite holidays for disabled people and carers.
0303 303 0145
www.revitalise.org.uk

Royal College of General Practitioners
Central body for general practitioners of medicine in the UK.
www.rcgp.org.uk

Royal College of Occupational Therapists
Find an occupational therapist.
020 7357 6480
www.rcot.co.uk

Royal Voluntary Society
Volunteer or get help for your loved ones.
www.royalvoluntaryservice.org.uk

St John Ambulance
First Aid courses.
www.sja.org.uk

Samaritans
If something is troubling you or your relative in any way, they will offer confidential help.
116 123
24 hours a day
www.samaritans.org

Senior Railcard
Discounts on train travel.
www.senior-railcard.co.uk

Tell Us Once
Register a death with various parties with one notification.
www.gov.uk/after-a-death/organisations-you-need-to-contact-and-tell-us-once

The Silver Line
A helpline offering support and a listening ear for older people.
0800 470 8090
24 hours a day
www.thesilverline.org.uk

Society of Later Life Advisers (SOLLA)
Find a financial adviser who specialises in helping older people.
https://societyoflaterlifeadvisers.co.uk

Stroke Association
Help and support after stroke.
020 7566 0300
www.stroke.org.uk

UK Funerals
Find a funeral director.
www.uk-funerals.co.uk

UK Gout Society
Information for those suffering with gout.
www.ukgoutsociety.org

United Kingdom Homecare Association
Help and advice on finding homecare.
0208 661 8188
www.ukhca.co.uk

University of the Third Age (U3A)
Learning for older people.
020 8466 6139
www.u3a.org.uk

Uswitch.com
Compares energy providers and helps you help your relative switch.
0800 6888 557
Mon–Fri 8 a.m.–9 p.m.; Sat 9 a.m.–5 p.m.; Sun 10 a.m.–4 p.m.
www.uswitch.com

Warm Home Discount Scheme Helpline
Informs you about discounts and benefits for which your relative might be eligible.
0345 603 9439
Mon–Fri 8.30 a.m.–4.30 p.m.
www.gov.uk/the-warm-home-discount-scheme

Acknowledgements

Writing this book has entailed enormous amounts of research and I would like to thank and acknowledge the following people and resources:

Carers Trust, www.gov.uk, www.lgo.org.uk, Age UK, Citizens Advice, HMRC, Society of Later Life Advisers (SOLLA), www.nhs.uk, Pension Wise, Money Advice Service, UKHCA, CQC, Julia Hart, Stella Nash, Sammy Margo, Alan Nevies, Gary Tatham, www.cot.co.uk, The Reiki Association, British Heart Foundation, Royal Voluntary Service, Arthritis Care, Arthritis Research UK, Bowel Cancer UK, Beating Bowel Cancer, Bladder & Bowel Community, Julian Kurer, Diabetes UK, Anchal Prasher, Parkinson's UK, Prostate Cancer UK, Stroke Association, Rebecca Penzer, Dementia UK, Alzheimer's Society, Alzheimer's Research UK, Anxiety UK, Mind, Huntington's Disease Association, Dying Matters and the National Association of Funeral Directors.

I would also like to thank my husband, two sons and George Stone.

Index